David L Dawson & Nima G Moghaddam

Formulation in Action. Applying Psychological Theory to Clinical Practice

David L Dawson & Nima G Moghaddam

Formulation in Action

Applying Psychological Theory to Clinical Practice

Managing Editor: Aneta Przepiórka

DE GRUYTER
OPEN

Published by De Gruyter Open Ltd, Warsaw/Berlin

ISBN: 978-3-11-047099-4
e-ISBN: 978-3-11-047101-4

Bibliographic information published by the Deutsche Nationalbibliothek.
The Deutsche Nationalbibliothek lists this publication in the Deutsche Nationalbibliografie; detailed bibliographic data are available in the Internet at http://dnb.dnb.de.

Managing Editor: Aneta Przepiórka

www.degruyteropen.com
Cover illustration: © YasnaTen

Contents

List of contributing authors

David L Dawson
University of Lincoln, UK
Chapters 1, 2, 3, 4

Nima G Moghaddam
University of Lincoln, UK
Chapters 1, 2, 3, 4

Ray St Ledger
Humber NHS Foundation Trust, UK
Chapter 3

David M Gresswell
University of Lincoln, UK
Chapters 3, 4, 9, 11

Aidan J P Hart
University of Lincoln, UK
Chapters 5, 6

Kerry Beckley
Lincolnshire Partnership NHS Foundation Trust, UK
Chapters 5, 6

Thomas Schröder
The University of Nottingham, UK
Chapters 7, 8

Angela Cooper
The Centre for Emotions and Health, Canada
Chapters 7, 8

Rohan Naidoo
Compass Wellbeing, UK
Chapters 7, 8

Anna Tickle
The University of Nottingham / Nottinghamshire Healthcare NHS Foundation Trust, UK
Chapters 7, 8

Michael Rennoldson
Nottingham Trent University, UK
Chapters 7, 8

Rachel Sabin-Farrell
The University of Nottingham / Nottinghamshire Healthcare NHS Foundation Trust, UK
Chapters 3, 9

Roger Bretherton
University of Lincoln, UK
Chapters 3, 9

Vanessa Dale-Hewitt
The University of Nottingham, UK
Chapter 10

Chris Irons
The Compassionate Mind Foundation, UK
Chapter 10

Louise Braham
The University of Nottingham / Nottinghamshire Healthcare NHS Foundation Trust, UK
Chapters 10, 11

Sharron Smith
University of Lincoln, UK
Chapters 10, 11

Danielle De Boos
The University of Nottingham, UK
Chapter 11

Acknowledgments

We would like to thank the contributors for their engagement with the project and for offering up their clinical work for critical evaluation. Special thanks to MG and Amou Meherdad for their influence over the years.

David L Dawson & Nima G Moghaddam

1 Formulation in Action: An Introduction

Every individual experiences a complex array of events, situations, and circumstances within their lifetime that influence their psychological development and sense of personhood. Previous relationships and attachments, social roles and expectations, formative experiences and contexts, education, gender, culture, and countless other factors influence how we perceive ourselves, the world, and those around us. The nexus between our personal characteristics and experiences is where our individuality and relationality lie, and – from a psychological perspective – our preferences, biases, behaviours, peccadillos, hopes, and fears are forged within this complex milieu.

Psychological formulation (and its derivatives: case formulation and case conceptualisation) is the dynamic framework used by many psychological practitioners, in a range of applied contexts, to manage and understand this complexity. While operational definitions vary subtly between different theoretical approaches, formulation in mental health settings can be broadly understood as the process – and product – of applying psychological theory and concepts to understand the aetiology, meaning, and maintenance of the psychological difficulties we, and others, experience, and to identify ways in which these difficulties may be managed (see Corrie & Lane, 2010; Johnstone & Dallos, 2013, for a comprehensive overview of definitions).

When individuals seek psychological support, formulation helps to guide identification of the processes, mechanisms, patterns, and so forth that appear to be contributing to the individual's difficulties, assisting the psychological practitioner – and the individuals they are engaged with – to look *through* the complexity in order to recognise the latent factors and processes that appear key to understanding the distress and its maintenance. In this way, formulation can be thought of as the process of looking past the ripples and waves in order to understand the underlying currents and how best to navigate or harness them. Formulation is therefore considered central to the role of many applied psychological practitioners (e.g., American Psychological Association, 2005; Division of Clinical Psychology, 2010), facilitating the idiographic application of established psychological principles, and thus providing the essential bridge between psychological theory and clinical practice (e.g., Butler, 1998; Division of Clinical Psychology, 2010; Kuyken, Fothergill, Musa, & Chadwick, 2005). Figure 1.1 below depicts how formulation is informed by both inductive (information that is specific to the client) and deductive (broader psychological theory) processes. Importantly, there is a reciprocal influence between client-specific information and how a theoretical framework is applied, enabling idiographic responsivity (Persons, 2008).

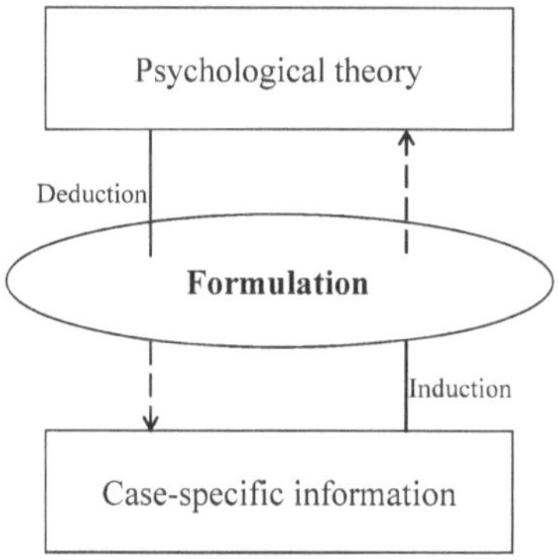

Figure 1.1: In principle, formulation is constructed, validated, and adjusted through ongoing processes of deduction (drawing from, and applying, theory) and induction (grounded in data). Dashed lines indicate that theory informs assessment of case-specific information, and case information informs how theory is applied. Through case-based abstractions, case information also has potential to inform theory-building. While the above represents an idealised model of the reciprocal relationship between theory and practice, idiographic practitioner factors (e.g., experience, biases, etc.) are likely to influence *how* theory is deduced and applied in practice

The theoretical landscape that underpins applied psychology and therapy is constantly developing and evolving, informed by advances in basic theory, clinical observation, research, data, politics, and fashion; and individual practitioners are trained and embed their practice within different theoretical schools, traditions, and models. The process of formulating, or 'applying theory to practice' within a discipline as diverse, critical, and factional as applied psychology can therefore often seem unclear – particularly to students and trainees who are developing their own competencies in this area and who might be anxious to ensure that they apply the 'right' theory 'correctly'. It is this process of applying psychological theory to clinical practice that is the central interest of the current volume.

The current volume has a strong applied focus and aims to demonstrate how a single case presentation ('Molly' – described in Chapter 2) can be formulated from a variety of theoretical perspectives. A single case description cannot capture the complexity, diversity, and dynamic processes of real-word clinical practice. However, by conveying multiple conceptualisations of a single client presentation, the salient features and unique aspects of each particular approach become more apparent – thus facilitating direct comparison and contrast between applied approaches. In this way, we wanted chapter contributors to illustrate *how* they apply psychological theory to their clinical practice, and to show their 'working out' – highlighting their initial thoughts and hypotheses, the case factors they consider salient and why, and how these issues sit within their approach – demonstrating 'formulation in action'.

Given the issues related to applying the 'right' theory 'correctly', outlined above and elsewhere (e.g., Eells, 2011; Sturmey & McMurran, 2011), we also wanted to stimulate a critical dialogue between psychological practitioners of different theoretical positions. In this way, we aimed to further augment the compare-and-contrast function of each chapter, but also to demonstrate that *all* psychological formulations are open to critique – that the process of focussing on specific, theory-aligned factors within a case will inevitably entail the holding or over-looking of others – and to evince the multiple perspectives that practitioners have and how these can be debated.

There are a number of very useful resources currently available that critically examine the nature, function, validity, reliability, and utility of formulation within applied psychology (e.g., Bruch, 2015; Corrie & Lane, 2010; Eells, 2011; Eells, Lombart, Kendjelic, Turner, & Lucas, 2005; Flinn, Braham, & Nair, 2014; Johnstone & Dallos, 2013), consider its role within the profession more broadly (e.g., as an alternative to psychiatric diagnosis; Division of Clinical Psychology, 2013; Johnstone & Dallos, 2013), and demonstrate how various cases may be conceptualised from different perspectives (e.g., Sturmey, 2009). While individual chapter contributors address some of these broader issues, the current volume aims to build on the strengths of these existing resources by focussing on the applied and critical aspects of psychological formulation in action.

1.1 The Current Volume

Recent estimates indicate that there are now over 400 psychotherapy models, with varying levels of evidential support (Wedding & Corsini, 2013). The current volume describes a selection of psychological approaches commonly employed in contemporary clinical practice. This selection reflects broader trends over recent decades within psychological practice in that, further to more established 'pure form' models (e.g., behavioural, cognitive, and psychodynamic approaches), it includes a number of integrative and hybrid approaches that 'build on' aspects of these traditional models. Approximately one third of practitioner psychologists now identify their primary 'theoretical' orientation as 'eclectic' or 'integrative' (Prochaska & Norcross, 2010) – suggesting that the adherence to 'pure form' models is losing ground to a more pragmatic, intermixed approach to therapy. While pragmatic approaches may allow for flexible application of evidence-based techniques according to the needs of individual cases, this may come at the expense of testability, depth, clarity, coherence, and theory development (Gilbert & Orlans, 2011). Similarly, when new approaches are developed that appropriate and incorporate empirically-established principles and techniques, it can become very difficult to discern whether the therapy is effective because of the new or old components, or a combination of both – compounding existing difficulties in identifying theory-specific versus common mechanisms of effective therapy. The current volume attempts to capture these tensions through the inclusion of traditional, contemporary, and integrative therapeutic approaches, and by eliciting critical dialogues between advocates of each.

1.2 Chapter Structure

1.2.1 Model Overview and Application

Chapter contributors were asked to provide an overview of their particular theoretical approach – highlighting the origins, central tenets, key principles, evidence for effectiveness, and common criticisms that are made of the approach – before proceeding to apply their specific theoretical approach to the case material presented in Chapter 2.

In these sections, the contributors were encouraged to show their 'working out' or 'formulation in action': demonstrating their initial understanding of the information provided, highlighting the issues that – from their theoretical position – are immediately salient and form key foci, and explicating how formulation interacts with these factors and processes. Finally, contributors were asked to outline potential intervention objectives, how these are underpinned by their theoretical approach, and how intervention effectiveness would be determined – a key area of debate within applied psychology settings.

1.2.2 Critical Commentary and Author Response

In order to foster debate and to highlight how particular approaches to formulation and therapy may be critiqued, we invited contributors of other theoretically-aligned chapters within the volume to critique the formulation and theoretical approach outlined in each chapter. To maximise variability, we aimed to pair psychological approaches that – at a theoretical level – should offer the most distinct contrasts: for example, pairing Intensive Short-term Dynamic Psychotherapy (hypothesising intrapsychic mechanisms of change) with Systemic Family Therapy (largely hypothesising extrapsychic mechanisms of change). These commentaries are designed to demonstrate the advantages, disadvantages, and broader issues with respect to adoption of any particular approach to formulation and therapy. Finally, all contributors were provided with a 'right to reply' in order to address, where possible, the issues raised in the critical commentary, and to reflect more broadly on issues of theoretical similarity and dissimilarity.

As editors, one of our primary aims has been to stimulate critical consideration and debate in relation to how psychological theory is applied in clinical practice. In addition to the issues highlighted and addressed within the critical commentaries, a number of authors have recommended criteria for the evaluation of applied theories (Cramer, 2013; Patterson, 1983; Prochaska, Wright, & Velicer, 2008; Sharf, 2015) – and we consider that these are applicable to both the (general) psychological models and (specific) formulations outlined in each chapter (although the relative importance of individual criteria may be considered to vary according to the epistemological positioning of each approach). The box below provides a synthesis of some of these criteria and associated questions: We recommend that readers hold these in mind when critically appraising case formulations and the psychological theories from which they are derived – both within this volume and in their own clinical practice.

Criterion	Indicator questions
Clarity and Parsimony	• Is the model understandable and internally consistent? • Is the model needlessly complex or convoluted? • Are key concepts discrete, specific, and non-redundant?
Precision and Testability	• Are concepts operationally defined and measurable? • Is the model too broad to have explanatory precision? • Does the model produce testable hypotheses? • Are propositions and inferences falsifiable? • Does the model allow for the clinician's assumptions to be disconfirmed?
Empirical adequacy	• Can the model account for available evidence? • Are model-based predictions demonstrably accurate? • Are the posited mechanisms or processes within the model empirically validated?
Comprehensiveness and Generalisability	• Is the model holistic? • Does the model apply across a range of contexts and clinical phenomena? • Does the model transfer to different situations and occasions?
Utility and Applied value	• Does the model provide a useful conceptual or heuristic framework for practice? • Does it facilitate shared understanding and workability? • Do interventions based on the model demonstrate effectiveness?

References

American Psychological Association. (2005). Report of the 2005 Presidential Task Force on Evidence-Based Practice. Washington, DC: APA.

Bruch, M. (2015). *Beyond diagnosis: Case formulation in cognitive behavioural therapy*. Chichester, UK: John Wiley & Sons.

Butler, G. (1998). Clinical formulation. In A. S. Bellack & M. E. Hersen (Eds.), *Comprehensive Clinical Psychology* (pp. 1-23). New York: Pergamon Press.

Corrie, S., & Lane, D. A. (2010). *Constructing stories, telling tales: A guide to formulation in applied psychology*. London: Karnac.

Cramer, K. M. (2013). Six criteria of a viable theory: Putting reversal theory to the test. *Journal of Motivation, Emotion, and Personality, 1*(1), 9-16.

Division of Clinical Psychology. (2010). *Clinical psychology: The core purpose and philosophy of the profession*. Leicester, UK: British Psychological Society.

Division of Clinical Psychology. (2013). Classification of behaviour and experience in relation to functional psychiatric diagnoses: Time for a paradigm shift. Leicester, UK: British Psychological Society.

Eells, T. D. (2011). *Handbook of psychotherapy case formulation*. New York: Guilford Press.

Eells, T. D., Lombart, K. G., Kendjelic, E. M., Turner, L. C., & Lucas, C. P. (2005). The quality of psychotherapy case formulations: a comparison of expert, experienced, and novice cognitive-behavioral and psychodynamic therapists. *Journal of Consulting and Clinical Psychology, 73*(4), 579-589.

Flinn, L., Braham, L., & Nair, R. d. (2014). How reliable are case formulations? A systematic literature review. *British Journal of Clinical Psychology*, Advance online publication. doi: 10.1111/bjc.12073

Gilbert, M., & Orlans, V. (2011). *Integrative therapy: 100 key points and techniques*. Hove: Routledge.

Johnstone, L., & Dallos, R. (2013). *Formulation in psychology and psychotherapy: Making sense of people's problems*. Hove: Routledge.

Kuyken, W., Fothergill, C. D., Musa, M., & Chadwick, P. (2005). The reliability and quality of cognitive case formulation. *Behaviour Research and Therapy, 43*(9), 1187-1201.

Patterson, C. H. (1983). *Theories of counseling and psychotherapy*. Philadelphia: Harper & Row.

Persons, J. B. (2008). *The case formulation approach to cognitive-behavior therapy*. New York: Guilford Press.

Prochaska, J. O., & Norcross, J. C. (2010). *Systems of psychotherapy: A transtheoretical analysis* (7th ed.). Pacific Grove, CA: Brooks/Cole.

Prochaska, J. O., Wright, J. A., & Velicer, W. F. (2008). Evaluating theories of health behavior change: A hierarchy of criteria applied to the transtheoretical model. *Applied Psychology, 57*(4), 561-588.

Sharf, R. (2015). *Theories of psychotherapy & counseling: Concepts and cases*. Boston, MA: Cengage Learning.

Sturmey, P. (2009). *Clinical case formulation: Varieties of approaches*. Chichester, UK: John Wiley & Sons.

Sturmey, P., & McMurran, M. (2011). *Forensic case formulation*. Chichester, UK: John Wiley & Sons.

Wedding, D., & Corsini, R. J. (2013). *Current Psychotherapies* (10th ed.). US: Brooks/Cole.

David L Dawson & Nima G Moghaddam

2 Case Description

The following case description provides the base material for each of the clinical case formulations in subsequent chapters. An overview of the client's history, experiences, and current circumstances is provided in a chronological, narrative form. Given that different psychological approaches prioritise, highlight, and attend to specific factors and client experiences differentially, we attempted to avoid imposing a structured, theoretically-aligned format on our contributors in order that their subsequent formulations could be aligned with their own ways of working. Direct quotations from the client are provided in quotation marks and provide insight into her own perceptions of her experiences and difficulties.

2.1 Introducing Molly

Molly is a 29-year old single woman who currently lives alone in a new, modest, rented apartment close to the city centre. Although she has one long-term close friend (Eve), and a number of casual acquaintances, she tends not to socialise a great deal as she finds it "difficult to be (herself) in larger groups". Instead, she uses social media to keep up with people and will talk to Eve on the telephone once every week or so. Molly works 30 hours a week at the city library close to her home, and until recently, enjoyed her job.

In her spare time, Molly likes to read, watch TV, cook, and browse online shops and auction websites for antique porcelain dolls. She also runs errands for her parents who live nearby, and although they are relatively young, Molly feels that they make excessive demands on her time and can make her feel guilty if she does not meet those demands.

2.1.1 Childhood and Early Adolescence

Molly has one younger sister, Ella, who is currently studying for a PhD at university. Although Molly is very close to Ella and has always relied on her for support, she feels that life has been easier for her sister and that their parents "love Ella more than (her)". Molly feels that Ella was "spoiled" as the youngest child and did not have to try as hard to earn their parents' affection.

Molly feels that her home life "lacked warmth" when she was growing up. Her parents lived quite separate lives within the same household; each had their own bedroom and sitting room where they would spend most of their time, but although Molly's mother would be verbally critical and dismissive of her father, there were no direct confrontations. In contrast, Molly was considered “overly emotional” and “dramatic” by her parents as she would become tearful and would fight with her sister over “little things”.

In contrast to other family members, Molly also had more contact with the family GP, frequently complaining of nausea and constipation. More recently, Molly was diagnosed with idiopathic pelvic pain and Irritable Bowel Syndrome (IBS).

At school, Molly was well-liked by her teachers but found it difficult to form and maintain relationships with the other children. She describes herself as being “too controlling” and “emotionally demanding” of the few friends she had, although “one or two girls put up with (her)”. Molly’s mother had high academic expectations and conveyed that Molly should be able achieve without relying on help from others; at times when Molly did not achieve as well as expected, her mother would express her disappointment by “giving one of her ‘looks’”.

2.1.2 Early Adulthood

From a young age Molly had always wanted to train as a teacher. She achieved good grades in her exams at school and college, and successfully obtained a teacher training position at university. However, although she was initially excited about starting university, the training programme involved many role-plays, presentations, and class discussions which made Molly feel “stressed” and “exposed”, and she began to avoid classes and assignments that involved direct participation. Consequently, she started to fall behind with her work, became less integrated with her peers in class, and due to her absences, was not invited to as many social occasions as other people.

Molly’s move to university was the first time she had been away from home for an extended period and she initially found not living with her parents difficult; although her fellow students seemed to embrace the freedom that university life offered, Molly found the experience somewhat overwhelming. However, her housemates were friendly and would cook, eat, and socialise together, but Molly would only join them if she was asked directly because she did not want to “impose” on the group.

One of the housemates, Jack, showed an interest in Molly, and after spending an afternoon drinking together, they went to Molly’s room to have sex. During the encounter, three other housemates charged into Molly’s room and teased the couple for being in bed together; although Jack laughed along with them, Molly felt acutely embarrassed and ashamed.

After her encounter with Jack, Molly tried to spend more time with him over the next month, but he appeared not to be interested in her anymore and accused her of being “clingy”; Molly believed he was purposefully ignoring her, was speaking badly about her to others, and “laughing” behind her back. Consequently, Molly began to withdraw further, and during her second term, dropped out of university altogether and returned home to live with her parents.

2.1.3 Adulthood

After leaving university, Molly worked various temporary jobs, mainly in administrative support and general office work. Although she obtained a position as a classroom assistant, this was a temporary position and the contract was not extended further. Molly felt that if she had "fitted in more" with the teachers and other staff members then perhaps they would have made her a fulltime member of staff.

After her period at university Molly lived intermittently with her parents until she was 27. During that time, she also lived briefly with a boyfriend (Danny) and her sister Ella. Although Molly and Ella lived together for a year and spent a lot of time together, they would frequently argue because Molly felt Ella had too many casual boyfriends, stayed out too often, and did not help enough around the house. When Ella was offered a funded PhD in another city, Molly returned to her parents' home as she could not afford the rent alone.

Molly's relationship with Danny was short-lived. Molly met Danny through a friend of her sister during a rare occasion when she had agreed to go out for a drink. Molly felt "very much in love" with Danny and was sure "he was the one", and moved into his flat with him around a month later. However, Danny ended the relationship the month after following an argument, telling Molly to move out of his flat, and accusing her of being "emotionally demanding" and of having moved in without "fully asking" him. Molly was devastated when Danny ended the relationship and felt ashamed at having to move back with her parents, particularly as they had told her that the relationship was "moving too fast" and would not last. A few weeks later, Molly discovered that Danny had been seeing other people when he was with Molly; shortly afterwards, Molly was admitted to hospital following an overdose of painkillers.

Molly was transferred to an acute psychiatric ward for two weeks. During that time she openly talked about feeling worthless, and nursing records report that Molly started to "copy" the behaviour of other individuals on the ward, including minor self-cutting, and that nursing staff felt Molly was "histrionic" and that her problems were "behavioural," "manipulative", "attention seeking", or due to a "personality disorder." However, other staff members felt they established a positive relationship with Molly and expressed sympathy that she did not receive any visitors during her admission.

Following discharge from hospital Molly returned to her parents' home. Although she had been advised to seek a referral for psychological therapy from her GP, Molly felt that any further contact with mental health services would add to the stigma her parents already felt by having a "daughter who had been in the madhouse". Molly felt that she "had to pull (herself) together" and that she had been "stupid to have such a reaction to a breakup with a boyfriend". She made extra effort with her parents, performing errands and chores for them, and obtained her job at the library after seeing the position advertised when returning some books for her mother.

After starting work, Molly moved out of her parents' home into her flat. She found her new independence markedly different from her time at university; she "enjoyed having a cleaning routine after work", became very "house proud", and started to enjoy baking cupcakes and brownies for her work colleagues.

More recently, another woman, Amy, started working at the library. When Amy first started, Molly "took her under (her) wing" and "showed her the ropes". The pair got on well for a month or so until Molly thought she heard Amy making a joke about Molly's clothes to another colleague. Molly did not confront Amy about the comment, but started to spend less time chatting with her colleagues and began to worry that they did not like her; she started to decline invitations for after-work drinks and stopped taking baked items to work.

2.1.4 Current Difficulties

Around this time, Molly started to have trouble sleeping; she would think about conversations she had had at work, what her colleagues had said to her, what she would have liked to have said to them, and would find it difficult to stop her "mind churning over the nonsense of the day". She would find it difficult to sleep and started staying up late during the week, often snacking and watching TV. Molly started to feel "constantly tired" at work, found it difficult to motivate herself to tidy her flat, felt she had little energy to do anything other than work and sleep, and previous hobbies gave her much less pleasure. Molly's weight also started to increase, and she would attempt to control this by not eating during the day, but would then feel very hungry in the evenings and would snack or order takeaway food.

Due to her sleeping difficulties, Molly requested help from her GP and was prescribed sleeping medication. However, although the medication helped Molly sleep, she found that she woke feeling very tired, remained lethargic throughout the day, and found it difficult to concentrate at work. In a further consultation with her GP, Molly reported that the medication was not helping her, that she was gaining weight, and that she often had "butterflies in (her) tummy" that frequently made her feel like she needed the toilet. After further prompts, Molly disclosed that she felt "miserable" and "stressed at work"; she became tearful and stated "there is no point in going on". She denied feeling suicidal but told her GP that she "just wanted help to sort (herself) out". After some initial protestation from Molly, her GP referred her for psychological therapy.

2.1.5 Psychological Therapy

Due to local demand for services, Molly was on the waiting list for psychological therapy for four months before she had an initial assessment. In her first session,

Molly appeared physically tense and sat very still and upright; her breathing was shallow and her gaze fluctuated markedly between the therapist and the door. She expressed anger at the therapist for having to wait so long to see someone, was confrontational and critical when the therapist attempted to explain the wait, and became overtly emotional – frequently sobbing and irritably snapping at some of the therapist's questions – but then apologising and expressing frustration for not "keeping (herself) together". Molly told the therapist that she felt "totally useless", and although she is "not stupid" she had "let everyone down" and felt that she had no real "role or importance to anyone special". Molly described her parents as "completely obsessed with themselves" and that they were "not really there" for her during her childhood. She told the therapist that "She [mum] would have loved to say I was a teacher" but that her parents must now see her as "a freak show".

Molly found her initial session with her therapist emotionally demanding but agreed to continue therapy; she has now had three sessions in total. As the sessions have progressed, Molly has told the therapist that she feels that she is underachieving at work, feels that others are losing patience and are critical of her, and that she is "weak and useless" because she is tearful and depressed. She refers to herself as "an irritation", "an embarrassment" and suggests that she has "never been enough" or "interesting".

In her second session, Molly alluded to "past traumas" but withheld from disclosing further information, instead stating that she "should be able to pull (herself) together and ought to be able to get on with things". However, in her most recent session, Molly disclosed that she was sexually abused when she was nine years old over a period of two months. She has never informed anyone of the experience, stating that her family would think she had "made up the allegations for attention", that it would "wreck the family", and that "you just have to get on with it". She presents as very reluctant to discuss the matter further.

Molly also informed her therapist that she believes Danny, her "first real boyfriend", finished their relationship because she was unable to be consistently sexually intimate with him. Although she reports having sexual thoughts and responses, and engages in occasional flirting, Molly worries about it "going too far" and feels "dirty" when she experiences a physical sexual response. She states that she feels "unattractive", "frumpy", and that she "couldn't believe that Danny had liked (her)" and that she is "not going to get that lucky again". She explains that there is "no point in having another relationship", because if she does not have sex with her partner, then he will "go elsewhere for it" and will "abandon (her) like Danny did". When telling her therapist this, she becomes visibly annoyed and states that she hates "being so needy".

2.1.6 Therapeutic Goals

Molly has found it difficult to clearly identify her goals for therapy. However, as the sessions have progressed, she has informed her therapist that she wants "to get better", "feel the opposite" of how she feels now, "feel more confident", and that she would "really like to make everyone proud in some way".

David L Dawson, David M Gresswell, Ray St Ledger & Nima G Moghaddam

3 Clinical Behaviour Analysis

Within this chapter, we formulate the case of Molly using the principles of Clinical Behaviour Analysis (CBA). At its core, CBA is the application of empirically established behavioural learning principles to the clinical domain, providing a framework for the systematic analysis of a person's historical and current contexts, in terms of the personal learning that has occurred through interaction with those contexts, and using this information to understand the function and maintenance of an individual's clinically-relevant behaviour.

Unlike other established approaches to formulation and therapy, CBA is often misunderstood by individuals who are unfamiliar, or only partially familiar, with the central tenets of the approach. Common charges levied against CBA (and its variants, such as applied behaviour analysis, 'behaviourism', 'behavioural approaches', etc.) include: the apparent dismissal of thoughts, feelings and emotions as unobservable and therefore unimportant to the clinician or analyst; the use of aversive techniques and punishment to change behaviour; and the reduction of the complexity of individual experience into simplistic behavioural units. While these criticisms may be valid for some forms of mechanistic behaviourism or misinformed individual therapists, they do not apply to the radical behaviourism of B F Skinner (Skinner, 1974) – the behavioural philosophy that underpins our approach.

3.1 Defining Features

The key principles of radical behaviourism are that behaviour is: (a) functional – that is, it serves a purpose within the context in which it arises; (b) elicited through the interaction of a person's specific biology, learning history, and current context; and (c) selected, shaped and maintained by the contextual consequences of the behaviour itself. Before examining these principles in closer detail, however, it is first important to define what is specifically meant by the term 'behaviour' within this approach.

From a radical behavioural perspective, *everything a person does is behaviour* and can be subject to a behavioural analysis. Some behaviour is conspicuous, overt, and observable, and this form of behaviour is perhaps most frequently considered the chief interest of behaviour analysts. However, radical behaviourism is also concerned with *private behaviours* – such as thinking, planning, and feeling – that are only available to the individual who is engaged in them. While it is accepted that such behaviours are difficult to observe and measure, such difficulties do not constitute a rationale for excluding them from a CBA:

> "Radical behaviourism...does not insist upon truth by agreement and can therefore consider events taking place in the private world within the skin. It does not call these events unobservable, and it does not dismiss them as subjective. It simply questions the nature of the object observed and the reliability of the observations" (Skinner, 1974, p. 17).

The classification of cognitions, emotions, and other interoceptive events as 'private behaviour' is more than a simple taxonomic sleight of hand, and alludes to one of the key defining features of radical behaviourism. Unlike other psychological theories, and more in line with the natural sciences, 'cognitions' – from this perspective, private verbal or visual behaviours – do not have *primacy*, and are thus classified as *dependent*, rather than *independent*, variables.

This demarcation is central to radical behaviourism and bears closer scrutiny. Within CBA, a holistic approach to the individual is adopted and cognitions and emotions are treated as important, complex responses (blends of overt, private, and physiological behaviour) that arise in a specific context; however, they are not the causes of the behaviour. An individual who experiences anxiety in a busy supermarket, for example, may experience visible signs of physiological arousal, and will likely experience private verbal behaviour with respect to the perceived threat ("I have to get out before something really bad happens to me"). However, within CBA, these experiences are *epiphenomenological* in the sense that they are the felt experience of interacting with a specific environmental context – they are not the cause of the anxiety, but a collection of complex *responses to* the supermarket as a contextual discriminative stimulus. Nonetheless, they are important responses – they provide the analyst with information regarding the personal meaning of particular stimuli (in terms of the learning that has previously taken place in relation to the stimuli), the salience of the stimuli (the strength and range of responses the stimuli elicit), and what consequences may be helping to maintain the behaviour (for example, escape behaviours may be maintained by resultant reductions in feelings of threat).

CBA therefore necessitates an idiographic, collaborative, and person-centred approach to therapy; the therapist is required to understand how an individual's unique learning experiences have led to the person's difficulties, and crucially, to understand how any therapeutic intervention may interact (favourably or unfavourably) with this prior learning. This emphasis on contextualising emotional experience is highly congruent with recent critiques of the Diagnostic and Statistical Manual of Mental Disorders (DSM) system (Brown & Gillard, 2015) which, given its structuralist underpinnings, tends to decontextualise difficulties and thus negate the personal meaning of the experience for the individual.

The key to understanding and working therapeutically with an individual within a CBA approach is through the production of a functional analysis – essentially a hypothesis (or series of hypotheses) about the acquisition, instigation, and maintenance of an individual's behaviour. The analyst aims to understand how an individual's learning history has led certain *antecedent* stimuli (such as events, interactions with others, verbal comments, etc.) to elicit specific *behaviours*, and how these behaviours, and different habits of approach and avoidance, have been shaped and maintained by their *consequences* through the mechanisms of reinforcement and punishment (outlined below). A functional analysis of a specific behaviour is therefore often delineated using a standard A:B:C: (antecedent, behaviour, consequences) framework. It is important to note the colons within the A:B:C: analysis: these serve to highlight that, as we are necessarily working with the retrospective recall of clients, we cannot always reliably determine that A caused B, and that B was maintained by C. However, we can establish that these events appear to follow each other in reliable ways, that changes in behaviour are consistent with learning theory principles, and that the analysis is congruent with current behaviour. In this way, functional analysis is underpinned by a pragmatic rather than positivistic epistemology (Biglan & Hayes, 1997).

In keeping with the scientific origins of CBA, the hypotheses generated about the maintenance of current behaviour should be both supported by the available data and testable (although this may not always be possible when analysing historic accounts of the acquisition of behaviours, as here). The ultimate goal of functional analysis from our perspective is to be able to predict and influence future behaviour with precision, scope, and depth (see Biglan & Hayes, 1997; Hayes, 1993).

3.2 Historical Origins and Key Principles

CBA is embedded in learning theory and can trace its origins to the late 19th and early 20th centuries, and the empirical work of Pavlov (1927; conditioned reflexes and classical conditioning); Thorndike (1931; trial and error learning and connectionism); Watson (1919; the formulation and fixation of habits and methodological behaviourism – specifically redefining psychology as the study of observable behaviour); and Skinner (1974; operant conditioning and radical behaviourism).

Within CBA, the primary interests of the analyst are the development of behaviour (through learning) and the function (rather than form or topography) of the behaviour (in terms of the consequences of the behaviour on the environment). The major learning theories that inform our approach are classical conditioning (often associated with Pavlov) and Skinner's operant conditioning. Although it is beyond the scope of this chapter to give a detailed account of the principles of classical and operant learning paradigms (see Pierce & Cheney, 2013, for an excellent overview) it is nevertheless necessary to articulate how we understand and use some of the key principles associated with these theories. At the simplest level, these approaches share the principle of temporal contiguity: Behaviours that are preceded by a stimulus can come to be elicited by that stimulus (classical conditioning), and behaviours that are followed by specific stimulus (consequence) can be reinforced and maintained by that stimulus (operant conditioning).

Many psychological models of clinical problems are in essence based on 'two factor theory' (e.g., Mowrer, 1956) in which clinically problematic behaviours initially develop through classical conditioning. An event – often something which induces fear or nausea, for example – becomes associated with a more neutral stimulus (such as a supermarket), and consequently, the supermarket comes to elicit a fearful or nausea-inducing learned response, in much the same way that a bell came to elicit salivation for Pavlov's dogs. However, unlike in Pavlov's original experiments with animals, when a neutral stimulus is associated with aversive, painful, or fear-inducing stimuli in humans, the association will often persist, and the strength of fearful response to the previously neutral stimulus may actually exceed the response to the original stimulus – a phenomenon known as "incubation" (Eysenck, 1968).

In two factor theory, however, the fearful behaviour is also maintained by operant processes. In operant theory, behaviours are effectively selected, shaped, and maintained by the influence they have on the environment; behaviours that have positive consequences for the individual, or which reduce the severity or probability of negative consequences, are maintained (reinforced), while those that are less effective in meeting their goals are reduced or abandoned (extinction). This process is analogous to the process of Darwinian natural selection, and Skinner highlighted the similarities between the environmental selection and shaping of biological processes at the level of the species, and the process of environmental selection and shaping of behaviours at the level of the individual within their own lifetime (Skinner, 1974).

Continuing our example above, if an individual experiences fear when entering a supermarket (possibly due to classical conditioning), that individual may leave the situation in an attempt to manage experienced anxiety; if this behaviour is successful and the individual's anxiety reduces, the avoidance/escape behaviour is likely to reoccur in the future – the behaviour has been negatively reinforced through the successful removal of the threat and will therefore be drawn upon again in similar circumstances.

Whereas reinforcement is defined as any consequence that increases the probability that a behaviour will reoccur in the future, *punishment* is the term given to any consequence that functions to reduce the likelihood of a behaviour recurring. However, in anything but extreme cases (such as immediate danger to life), and in line with Skinner's own views, punishment should have no place in therapy. Aside from the moral and ethical issues of using punishment within a therapeutic environment, such strategies generally function to merely suppress behaviour, often temporarily, rather than to eliminate it. Furthermore, by definition, punishment is experienced as highly aversive; can unintentionally result in other, undesired behaviours (such as anger or anxiety) becoming more salient; and only informs the punished individual about what *not* to do – it does not provide guidance or learning regarding what *to* do (i.e., punishment does not foster alternative functional behaviours):

> "In the long run, punishment, unlike reinforcement, works to the disadvantage of both the punished organism and the punishing agency. The aversive stimuli that are needed generate emotions, including predispositions to escape or retaliate, and disabling anxieties" (Skinner, 1953, p. 183).

Unfortunately, punishing behaviour can be very reinforcing for the punisher given that it can often result in immediate, albeit temporary, cessation of an unwanted behaviour, and perhaps explains why punishment can become part of the culture of any institution which has power and control over less-powerful individuals.

Due to common misunderstanding, however, it is important to note that reinforcement and punishment are *functionally* defined – they are defined by their effect on behaviour, *not* their topography. For example, public praise may act a positive reinforcer for one individual (it may increase a desirable behaviour by functioning as a 'reward'), but could function as a punisher for another individual (it may be experienced as embarrassing and decrease the likelihood of the targeted behaviour recurring). Similarly, what appears to be a punishing stimulus, such as the infliction of pain, may actually function as a reinforcer for some individuals in some contexts (e.g., individuals who enjoy masochistic sex practices).

In addition to reinforcement and punishment – the frequency and temporality of the delivery of such consequences (or 'schedule of reinforcement') is also crucial. Behaviours that are always reinforced in predictable ways are much easier to extinguish than behaviours that are subject to intermittent or unpredictable schedules of reinforcement – these latter schedules are very successful at maintaining behaviour over long periods, and are the types of schedules most frequently encountered by clinicians in the therapy room. A classic example of an intermittent schedule is found in gambling – the individual does not know how many times they need to gamble in order to win, and consequently, the gambling behaviour can be very resistant to extinction; the gambler may 'chase' losses, expecting reinforcement (winning) to occur at any time, and thus the behaviour continues.

Radical behaviourists also take full account of the role of language in learning and influencing behaviour; people are verbal beings living in a verbal community, and language can shape and influence behaviour by changing the abstract value and relative importance of stimuli and reinforcers, or by verbally specifying the consequences of a particular behaviour or course of action (termed 'rule governed behaviour' within radical behaviourism). In this way, individuals not only learn by direct experience (e.g., through direct contact with the environmental consequences of their own behaviour) but also through verbal means such as rules, instruction, and culture (Hayes, Barnes-Holmes, & Roche, 2001; Skinner, 1974).

Finally, within CBA, the analyst is also interested in the identification of behavioural conflicts which emerge through competing appetitive (positively reinforced) and/or aversive (negatively reinforced and/or punished) histories of reinforcement. Examples include: (1) approach/avoidance conflicts – 'I want to eat the chocolate bar (appetitive) but if I do I may put on weight (aversive)'; (2) avoidance/avoidance conflicts – 'I don't want to write this essay (aversive) but if I don't I may fail my course (aversive)'; and (3) approach/approach conflicts 'I want to go to the concert (appetitive) but I also want to stay at home and take a bath (appetitive)'. While these examples illustrate the phenomenon, more significant conflicts can result in stress, indecision, and important clinical presentations.

3.3 Empirical Evidence

The mechanisms underpinning behavioural approaches are amongst the most broadly applicable and empirically-supported in the whole of applied (and experimental) psychology. Strong evidence for the effectiveness of behavioural approaches to therapy can be found in a myriad of meta-analyses across a range of presentations and populations, including: depression (e.g., Cuijpers, van Straten, Andersson, & van Oppen, 2008; Cuijpers, Van Straten, & Warmerdam, 2007), anxiety disorders (e.g., Deacon & Abramowitz, 2004; Feske & Chambless, 1995; Kobak, Greist, Jefferson, Katzelnick, & Henk, 1998), autism (e.g., Eldevik et al., 2009), attention-deficit hyperactivity disorder (Fabiano et al., 2009), chronic pain (e.g., Morley, Eccleston, & Williams, 1999), insomnia (Smith et al., 2014) and many others (for an overview, see Kazdin, 2013). Indeed, Pierce and Cheney (2013) state that the principles underpinning behavioural approaches are so broadly applicable "because the world actually operates according to these principles" (p.399) and the effective components of other therapies are often found to be those that rely on behavioural principles (e.g., Weinberger & Rasco, 2007).

3.4 Critique

The approaches of Watson and other early methodological behaviourists, predicated on logical positivism, have historically been somewhat conflated with Skinner's radical behaviourism. This erroneous assumption has led to any approach using the term 'behaviourism', including radical behaviourism, to be seen as simplistic, mechanistic, punitive, and dismissive of the roles of language and cognition, regardless of Skinner's own writings to the contrary (e.g., Skinner, 1974, 1989). However, Skinner's early accounts of therapy, language, and verbal behaviour are certainly not beyond critique, and Skinner's primary writings on these subjects (e.g., 1953, 1957) were initially based on extrapolations rather than solid data. However, radical behaviourism-informed approaches have continued to make significant data-driven advances in psychological theory and practice, leading to the development of Relational Frame Theory as a coherent behavioural account of language and cognition (Hayes et al., 2001), and radical behavioural-informed therapeutic approaches such as Acceptance and Commitment Therapy (Hayes, Strosahl, & Wilson, 1999; see Chapter 5) and Functional Analytic Psychotherapy (Kohlenberg & Tsai, 1991).

In addition to the general criticisms of radical behaviourism as a model of human functioning, negative perceptions of behavioural approaches are found amongst clinicians, healthcare professionals, and the general public more broadly. These appear to arise for a number of reasons:

1. Behavioural approaches have good 'common sense' face validity and can therefore appear both simplistic and mechanistic. Consequently, inexperienced practitioners can assume an expertise on the basis of very limited basic training, understanding, and supervision, leading to problematic and non-person-centred delivery of the approach with clients.
2. Behavioural approaches are very effective at reducing clinical behaviours when correctly applied, but if misapplied, can result in a strengthening of those behaviours or the development of other problematic behaviours.
3. Within some settings, inexperienced and poorly supervised healthcare professionals have at times developed 'behavioural programmes' based almost exclusively on punishment schedules that are highly reinforcing for staff members – they change behaviour quickly within the short-term – at the expense of a positive, helpful, and therapeutic experience for the client.
4. The term 'behavioural' has become somewhat of a stigmatising term when applied to clients by some healthcare professionals, where presentations or difficulties that seem purposeful are dismissed as 'behavioural' (deliberate), with the erroneous implication that these behaviours require less understanding or intervention.

Given that few other psychological approaches are as consistent as radical behaviourism with the scientist-practitioner philosophy prevalent in modern clinical psychology, or are as holistic in their attempts to balance all of the components of human experience (including emphasising the role of context), why have these criticisms remained? Skinner (1974) observed that the person with whom we are most familiar is our self and, before we come to study psychology, we typically have many years of being reinforced for explaining our own behaviour in terms of mental and emotional causes: change is often difficult, even for psychologists.

3.5 Formulation in Action

When working with Molly from a CBA perspective, our assessment would focus on (1) developing a functional analysis/formulation of her current behaviour (including private behaviour) in relation to her specific learning history (e.g., exploring what behaviours have been conditioned, reinforced, punished, and shaped historically); and (2) examining the function and consequences of her current behaviour in relation to her reported difficulties and therapeutic goals. Given our functional underpinnings, the classification of Molly's behaviour in terms of diagnosis would not be a priority.

The case material provided already contains some of the information we would attempt to elicit during an assessment and we can therefore begin to make provisional hypotheses. However, the information provided does not facilitate the identification of discrete behavioural chains or provide us with a means to examine the specific consequences of what appear to be key learning events. This somewhat precludes a traditional A:B:C: analysis, and consequently our formulation is tentative and the analysis provisional. In contrast to our usual clinical practice, wherein we would work with the client to refine the analysis, the formulation presented below is necessarily somewhat assumptive and accordingly loses some precision.

3.5.1 Initial Formulation

The working hypotheses outlined below are based on our reading and abstraction of events from Molly's self-report and presentation within therapy. We identified a number of areas that appear to be adversely impacting on Molly and would aim to explore these further in line with her therapeutic goals (see *intervention objectives* below). We have clustered these into three broad domains: (1) sex and relationships; (2) depression; and (3) social interaction. Given that we are unable to undertake a comprehensive functional analysis without further detailed information, we examine each of these domains in turn utilising a narrative framework (based on behavioural principles) to highlight salient events, learning, and behavioural mechanisms that appear relevant to understanding how Molly's difficulties may have developed.

3.5.1.1 Sex and Relationships

There is evidence from Molly's self-report that she may be experiencing difficulties with respect to her sexual functioning, and her ability and willingness to form and sustain relationships. Regarding sex, Molly reports feeling "dirty" when experiencing a sexual response, worries that if she doesn't have sex with a partner they will leave her, intimates that she is "not going to get that lucky again" (in finding a partner), but also worries about sexual encounters "going too far". Sexual stimulation and access to intimate partners are typically strong appetitive reinforcers and are important aspects of psychological wellbeing (e.g., Laumann et al., 2006; Laumann, Paik, & Rosen, 1999). However, in Molly's case, her history of rejection and humiliation within sexual relationships (such as her encounter with Jack at university) appears to have led to sexual activity becoming associated (conditioned) with aversive consequences.

Most of Molly's familial and social relationships appear to have been similarly marked by disappointment, rejection, and potential abuse, incrementally consolidating learning that relationships are generally difficult and hurtful. We would therefore hypothesise that these experiences have led to the development of a significant approach/avoidance conflict: meaningful relationships and intimacy are strongly desired but are unsafe and to be avoided.

3.5.1.2 Depression

Molly's self-report contains numerous references to low mood and factors commonly associated with 'depression'[1]. She is tearful and tense in her sessions with the therapist, she discloses feeling "miserable", "useless", "depressed", and "unattractive" – among other negative self-evaluations – and reports sleep disturbance, poor motivation, poor concentration, changed eating habits, and a lack of pleasure in previously enjoyed activities.

From a behavioural perspective, an individual experiences depression when a significant reduction in response-contingent positive reinforcement occurs, such as separation from a long-term partner, or as their behaviour becomes subject to increasing levels of aversive control (e.g., Ferster, 1973; Lewinsohn, 1974), such as having to perform excessive duties to avoid negative consequences (see Kanter, Busch, Weeks, & Landes, 2008, for an overview). Although most people will experience such changes in contingencies periodically within their lifetime, for some individuals, depressive behaviour can become more entrenched. This may occur through a lack of established adaptive behaviours that can help an individual to re-establish positive contingencies (such as social skills – see below), or through excessive avoidance behaviour, which functions to reduce imminent distress but at the cost of reducing the probability of contact with future sources of positive reinforcement.

Molly's avoidance of relationships is reducing her access to a number of strong primary reinforcers, such as sex, love, intimacy, social support, and safety. We would hypothesise that the series of events Molly has reported (and others which she has not yet reported) have led to a reduction in response-contingent reinforcement: many previous sources of positive reinforcement (such as work, baking, socialising with work colleagues, etc.) have subsequently become punishing through their association with humiliation, rejection, and failure. As a consequence, instead of actively approaching aversive situations or managing conflicts, Molly avoids activities and opportunities that may lead to positive reinforcement (such as socialising) in order to reduce potential near-term distress; this functions to maintain her behaviour through the mechanism of negative reinforcement.

1 We use 'depression' cautiously here as an umbrella term for a number of behaviours (overt and private) that commonly occur together when an individual is poorly reinforced by their environment. Within a behavioural analysis, depression is not something a person 'has' that *causes* these behaviours, but is simply a shorthand term *for* those behaviours.

Much of Molly's current and historical behavioural activity also appears under aversive control: her academic achievements, and university and career ambitions, appear to function to reduce her parent's "disappointment" rather than being aligned with her own personal values, and she reports running errands and meeting her parent's "excessive demands" in order to assuage feelings of guilt. Aside from contributing to low mood, another common consequence of such aversive schedules of reinforcement is anger and frustration, and there is evidence of both within Molly's self-report and therapeutic presentation. From a behavioural perspective, anger is typically considered to function as an energising/invigorating response to facilitate escape from an aversive environment, and Molly's occasional outbursts, both towards others and within therapy, provide us with important information about the dominance of negative reinforcement and punishment within her current context.

3.5.1.3 Social Interaction

There are indications from Molly's self-report and her presentation within therapy that she may have difficulties with social interactions. She describes herself as "too controlling" and "emotionally demanding" within most of her previous social and romantic relationships, and communicates feelings of social uncertainty (e.g., "not fitting in", not wanting to "impose" on other people at university, etc.). While Molly's difficulties in this domain may simply be bad luck (e.g., not meeting the right type of people), we would want to explore this further and have three (overlapping) tentative hypotheses at this stage:

(1) It is possible that Molly has not had sufficient opportunity to develop mature social interaction skills and her difficulties in this area may indicate a skills deficit. Some information within the case description is supportive of this hypothesis. Her parents do not appear to have modelled appropriate interaction behaviour – they are dismissive, avoidant, and critical of each other, and do not appear to have fostered sufficient "warmth" within the family home where the development (reinforcement) and refinement (shaping) of good social skills could occur. Similarly, any expression of need from Molly appears to have been labelled "dramatic", "clingy", and "histrionic" by her parents, partners, and even healthcare professionals during her hospital admission. These punishing consequences fail to provide Molly with opportunities to learn how to meet her needs in more socially acceptable ways and simply function to confirm her negative views of herself as an "irritation" and a "disappointment". Given that Molly's self-report indicates that her sister Ella *has* developed good social skills, however, we would want to examine this issue further: perhaps Ella was more favoured, or perhaps the alleged abuse is an important consideration here.

(2) Given Molly's reported history, we would also hypothesise that she has developed a need to tightly control the parameters of her relationships. She describes being "too controlling" and "emotionally demanding", and her behaviour in this regard – if these descriptions are accurate – may function as an attempt to minimise the

probability of harm (punishment) from potential relationships. Given that almost all of the relationships Molly has disclosed have resulted in distressing consequences for her (conditioned association), "clingy" and "controlling" behaviours are perhaps being maintained through perceived threat reduction – the more she controls her relationships, the more in control and less threatened she feels (negative reinforcement). However, the undesirable consequence of her controlling behaviour is that her relationships are more likely to breakdown given her difficult behaviour within them; this leads to the eventual removal of strong appetitive reinforcers (likely to contribute to low mood) and maintains (through a strong intermittent negative reinforcement schedule) her controlling behaviour in future relationships.

(3) Related to the above hypotheses, we would also want to explore the function of Molly's self-report and presentation during therapy. When first encountering Molly's history and the words she uses to describe herself, our first reactions are sympathy and compassion. However, while her report of her difficulties may well be accurate (and we would not aim to explore this further until a firm therapeutic relationship had been established), it may also be the case that the self-report itself, or more accurately, the *style* Molly uses to convey her history, is a prima facie indication of her social interaction difficulties. This is by no means to diminish Molly's distress, but her style of interaction may function to elicit sympathy and associated comfort from others, including the therapist. This would be congruent with the above hypotheses, perhaps suggesting limited skills for achieving intimacy in other, less demanding ways, and/or a behavioural style that aims to influence other people's emotional consideration towards her. While such an interaction style may be positively reinforced in the short-term, the long-term consequences may again be frustration and relationship breakdown as others start to consider Molly "emotionally demanding" and begin to avoid her: maintaining her problematic interaction style while also reducing her opportunities for long-term positive reinforcement through more subtle positive social interaction.

3.5.2 Intervention Objectives

When working with a client from within a CBA framework, our broad intervention objectives are: (1) to determine the nature and meaning of the client's therapeutic goals; (2) to establish the therapist and the therapeutic relationship as a robust source of positive reinforcement and a non-punishing context (this should occur at all stages of the assessment and intervention); (3) to undertake a detailed assessment leading to the production of an agreed formulation; (4) to use the formulation with the client to identify and understand helpful and unhelpful current behaviours (defined pragmatically as those that move the client closer to, or further away from, their therapeutic goals), and the reinforcement schedules that are maintaining or reducing them; and

(5) to develop with the client techniques, strategies, and behavioural experiments that facilitate therapeutic learning and behavioural change.

From a radical behavioural perspective, behaviour change (regardless of therapeutic modality) is effected through a limited number of processes. When working therapeutically with a client, we would therefore be guided by the principles that (1) desired behaviours are most successfully developed, shaped, and maintained through positive reinforcement (initially using a direct 1:1 ratio schedule where possible, before moving to intermittent ratios to ensure resilience); (2) problematic behaviours (those that have consequences that lead the client away from their therapeutic objectives) can be reduced through differential non-attendance on the part of the therapist when they occur, and can often be replaced through reinforcement of alternative behaviours that have a similar function (they meet the client's needs but without the previous negative consequences – termed *differential reinforcement of alternative behaviour*); (3) previously entrenched responses to specific stimuli, including those underpinned by rule-governed behaviour, can be disrupted and new learning take place through techniques such as structured exposure and desensitisation. Below, we describe how we would bring these elements together when working with Molly, the difficulties that may arise, and how we might assess the effectiveness of the intervention.

3.5.3 Intervention Plan

When working directly with clients we would always ensure that therapeutic goals are clearly stated in terms of measurable change, and would spend considerable time helping clients to identify and articulate these before beginning any intervention. We would use questions such as: 'if you were to achieve that goal, how would I know you had achieved it?'; 'how would other people know?'; 'if you managed to change that aspect of your life, what would you be doing differently?' The purpose of these types of questions is for the therapist and client to have a shared understanding of the *specific* nature of the behaviours the client wishes to change or develop, and importantly, provides a more concrete basis against which therapeutic gains can be evaluated.

Given Molly's history, we would expect her to have difficulties in specifying her therapeutic goals, and this seems to be the case; a great deal of her previous and current behaviour appears to have been orientated towards avoiding disapproval from others (negatively reinforced), and identifying goals for herself is likely to be relatively novel and therefore difficult. We would consequently spend time within initial sessions focussing Molly's attention on this issue, and using functional analysis to examine the *function* of her stated therapeutic goals: who are the desired changes for? What might the long-term consequences of those changes be? Are the changes likely to lead to more positive feedback from the environment, or just less negative feedback? Do the proposed changes look similar to previously problematic behaviour (in terms of function), or do they open up new possibilities?

Concurrently, we would also focus on building the formulation and developing the therapeutic relationship by positioning ourselves as a source of positive reinforcement and non-punishment. We would be attentive to and increase the types of comments, actions, and behaviours on our part that appeared to increase Molly's feelings of trust, safety, and openness, and would reduce behaviours (at the beginning of therapy) that had the opposite effect. Our behaviour here would again be based on function and not topography: for example, what we may consider a positive comment or behaviour may be experienced by Molly as condescending or dismissive. The therapist is therefore required to track the impact of their behaviour on the client to ensure that the therapeutic context is functioning to increase desired behaviour while reducing the frequency of undesired behaviour, in line with the client's therapeutic goals. From a behavioural perspective, everything that happens within the therapy room (including the therapist's own behaviour) can be subject to a functional analysis, and the negotiation of therapeutic goals and the development of the therapeutic relationship are no different.

As Molly became more comfortable within therapy (that is, following repeated experiences of direct response contingent positive reinforcement), we would begin to examine her history, presentation, and difficulties in closer detail, collaboratively building the formulation and developing functional analyses of her current behaviour. We would expect that Molly would become more tolerant of challenges from the therapist, given that such challenges, and her responses to them, would not necessitate withdrawal of positive reinforcement, and this initial foundation would be used to frame the whole therapeutic process.

It is important to note here that within CBA, the processes of assessment and formulation are not always clearly demarcated; what happens within the therapy room (and outside, during homework tasks and behavioural experiments) will impact on the formulation, more details are likely to be shared as the therapeutic relationship is developed, and the aims of therapy may change once understood within the context of the client's broader history. However, as noted above, before the principal intervention can proceed it is imperative that the client's therapeutic goals, and criteria for determining whether they have been achieved, are clearly established.

We cannot negotiate intervention targets directly with Molly and therefore we must make some assumptions regarding her therapeutic goals. Based on our provisional formulation, we would initially focus on Molly's social interaction and her depressive behaviour. We would expect that focussing on these components would have secondary benefits for the other domains of Molly's life (e.g. relationships) by providing her with skills to express and meet her needs in ways that are less problematic and that facilitate greater opportunity for positive reinforcement.

3.5.3.1 Social Interaction

We would use a combination of functional analysis, within-session interactions, and behavioural experiments to help Molly develop more adaptive social interaction behaviours. Using functional analysis, we would outline how certain events (such as comments from colleagues) appear to elicit specific behaviours (e.g., rumination, avoidance, etc.) and identify the consequences of these behaviours – in terms of whether they move Molly closer to, or further away from, the type of life she wishes to lead. We would hope to demonstrate to Molly that her behaviour (generally avoidance and isolation), although seemingly beneficial in the short-term, has significant long-term consequences for her. Through this process, we are attempting to undermine the learned associations and rule-governed behaviour that impact on Molly (e.g., 'the only way to cope with hurtful experiences is to avoid them') and to begin to introduce and reinforce alternative considerations (e.g., 'the cost of avoiding all difficult situations is having few friends and not being valued').

Using the therapeutic relationship as a basis of support, we would also strongly reinforce Molly's socially adaptive behaviour within the therapy session (such as appropriate, assertive expression of her needs; using more positive and less derogatory self-referential terms; challenging the therapist in an appropriate and socially skilled manner, etc.) and would attend less to any inappropriate (again, functionally defined, in terms of therapeutic goals) social behaviour. Although other approaches may refer to this process as 'non-specific factors', we would highlight the purposive use of differential reinforcement and shaping here to help develop Molly's social skills set.

Through the above, we would hope that Molly would begin to understand the potential (unintended) consequences of her previous interaction behaviours, to understand (at least in principle) that avoidance behaviours can have detrimental long-term consequences, and to have developed, through practice with the therapist, more adaptive ways of communicating her needs.

At this stage, we would want Molly to experience putting her new skills into practice, and would collaboratively develop behavioural exposure tasks for that purpose. Although the specific nature of the task would depend on Molly's therapeutic goals (for example, initiating a conversation with her work colleagues), the function of the task would be for Molly to experience direct, positive contingencies for her differential behaviour (in this case, tolerating rather than avoiding social discomfort), in order to promote and consolidate alternative, adaptive learning (in this case, through the process of exposure and habituation).

3.5.3.2 Depression

Behavioural activation is an effective behavioural approach for depression that aims to increase response-contingent positive reinforcement and reduce the occurrence of aversive control within an individual's life (Jacobson et al., 1996; Jacobson, Martell,

& Dimidjian, 2001; Martell, Addis, & Jacobson, 2001). Similar to the process of exposure for anxiety-related behaviours, 'activation' encourages individuals to engage in activities that they have been avoiding, in order to disrupt entrenched schedules of negative reinforcement and increase the opportunity for response-contingent positive reinforcement.

In line with behavioural activation, we would work with Molly to create a rank order of potentially reinforcing activities, and construct a schedule and structure for these activities (including planned frequency, intensity, and duration). Molly would then be encouraged to work through the agreed schedule between sessions, engaging in tasks in a graded manner (increasing activity over time, in order of task difficulty). Given that the aim of the procedure is to increase positive reinforcement and reduce aversive consequences, it is important that the tasks identified by the client are personally meaningful and are achievable. It is therefore judicious to start with readily-attainable, but personally salient tasks, so that the client has immediate experience of success, helping to maintain (positively reinforce) the approach behaviour for the remainder of the hierarchy, and consolidating learning. When engaging in a specified activity (for example, baking cakes for her colleagues again), Molly would be asked to rate each activity in terms of pleasure, mood, and mastery; these ratings would be discussed within subsequent therapy sessions, highlighting and reinforcing the relationship between activity and positive mood (and avoidance and negative mood).

We would expect that through the above interventions, Molly would become readily aware of the role of negative reinforcement in the maintenance of many of her difficulties; accordingly, we would expect Molly to become less avoidant and more approach-focussed in her response-style, and would therefore anticipate secondary positive effects in other areas of Molly's life that we have not directly targeted (such as her familial and sexual relationships).

3.5.3.3 Evaluation

The effectiveness of a behavioural intervention is determined pragmatically by whether the targeted behaviour(s) have significantly changed (e.g., increased or decreased) in line with the therapeutic goals established during the initial stages of therapy. To assess change in these behaviours, a combination of observation, self-report, and idiographic outcome measures are typically used, and the therapist may employ single-case methods (such as visual analysis of plotted data, reliable and clinical change statistics, etc.; Barlow, Nock, & Hersen, 2009; Hageman & Arrindell, 1999; Morley, 2013), in addition to the client's self-report, to ascertain intervention efficacy. Such methods allow for an idiographic but empirically-grounded approach to outcome assessment, and would underpin our work with Molly.

3.5.3.4 Potential Difficulties

Behaviour change is difficult, and it is likely that we would encounter a number of problems when initially working with Molly. Given her apparent tendency to avoid challenging situations (particularly social situations), her mistrust of relationships, her experiences of parental disapproval, and her possible limited social interaction skills, we would expect the beginning stages of therapy to be marked by a similar approach-avoidance style as her broader relationships. Consequently, frequent displays of emotion, followed by withdrawal and negative self-appraisals might be expected, as perhaps would be over-reporting on baseline measures of distress (given her limited ability, at that stage, to communicate her distress in other ways) – and this would need to be taken into account when attempting to measure therapy outcomes. We would aim to strike a balance between validating Molly's distress (in order to create a safe therapeutic space, to develop the therapeutic relationship, and to reduce the likelihood of premature therapy termination) and inadvertently reinforcing her problematic behaviours (making it more difficult to challenge those behaviours in the future). As therapy progressed, we would be optimistic that this gentle shaping process would reduce Molly's approach-avoidance conflict and would facilitate a strong, therapeutic relationship that would form the foundation for the above intervention.

Roger Bretherton & Rachel Sabin-Farrell

3.6 CBA Formulation: Critical Commentary

Reading the opening of this chapter was surprisingly pleasant, like taking a nostalgic trip down memory lane. Clinical Psychologists trained over the last few decades have been drilled and skilled in behavioural therapy and its derivatives as part of their training, and behavioural theory is therefore inseparable from the history and identity of Clinical Psychology in the UK. The principal hurdle to be overcome in critiquing this chapter is the strong sense of familiarity it is likely to induce in any Clinical Psychologist who reads it. In addition, more integrative approaches, such as Body-Centred Psychotherapy (see Chapter 9), openly acknowledge influences from behavioural theory among others.

It is therefore difficult to strongly assert that CBA is wrong *per se*. The early theoretical sections of the chapter state the principles of behavioural learning, most of which are undeniably true: we learn, animals learn, classically, operantly, two-factorly...and so on. But there is a point in this discourse where it turns from stating what is self-evidently true to what is unreflectively speculative. The main weakness of this chapter and the application of CBA to Molly's case is therefore not so much that the basic principles of CBA are wrong, but that they are overextended and narrow.

CBA bears all the marks of attempting to be a 'theory of everything' – a psychological approach, the basic principles of which can render a complete account of the essence of all human experience. 'Theories of everything' are closed and inflexible in their doctrines and therefore less open to development and consideration of new ideas. An approach such as CBA, as a theory of everything, not only has to demonstrate that it is clinically effective but it also has to show that other conceptualisations are not. Or, it has to account for the clinical effectiveness of other approaches by asserting that they are really just crypto-CBA – behaviourism in disguise. It therefore leans towards intolerance of alternative systems of thinking – an intolerance that will no doubt be demonstrated in the critique of our BCP chapter. Ironically, exclusive adherence to learning theory leads to a curious inability to learn from other theories.

In addition, while the writers of the CBA chapter are keen to stress that radical behaviourism is neither mechanistic nor reductive, simply stating the fact does not make it so. It seems likely that CBA at least qualifies as a *conceptually* reductive system of thought. CBA, it would appear, asserts that when push comes to shove, *everything* is behavioural contingency. Ultimately though, CBA is not an approach that allows any external critique. Skinner, it would appear, considered psychologists who detracted from behaviourism to be suffering the unfortunate consequences of having their introspective meanderings inappropriately reinforced. This is a good example of what social psychologists call an intra-textual hermeneutic, the way in which a social group closes itself to information outside of its borders – otherwise known as fundamentalism.

All of the above is likely to impact on the therapeutic practice offered by CBA. The central feature of which seems to be the excessive and unnecessary need to translate *everything* that happens into the language of behavioural contingencies. Take, for example, the description of Molly's growing comfort with the therapeutic situation. A behavioural account of this gradual acclimatisation to a novel environment is perfectly acceptable, but the language of relationship is surely much more appropriate to denote this development. Whereas other approaches would frame this in terms of increasing trust, rapport, collaboration, or empathy, the authors of this chapter prefer the heart-warming phrase, "repeated experiences of direct response contingent positive reinforcement", with the therapist a "source of positive reinforcement and non-punishment". The authors' reactions to Molly's history are "sympathy and compassion", but seemingly pathologise "her style of interaction" functioning to "elicit sympathy and associated comfort", with a "behavioural style that aims to influence other people's emotional consideration towards her". Surely this is a fundamental part of human to human interaction, so of course Molly's behaviour aims to influence other people in this way.

More hearteningly, later in the chapter, the phrase "a basis of support" is used to describe the therapeutic relationship. However, during therapy, the therapist would presumably decide which "socially adaptive behaviours" to reinforce and which "inappropriate" behaviours to attend less to. This represents a balance of power in favour of the therapist, which is further reinforced by phrases like "at this stage we would want Molly to...". It is acknowledged that there is likely to be difficulty in establishing goals, due to Molly avoiding disapproval from others. One wonders therefore how pressing on with specifying goals would seem to the client who is likely to want to avoid disapproval from the therapist, and how they would ensure that the goals were from the client and not imposed by the therapist. It is stated earlier in the chapter that there are professional and public negative perceptions of behavioural approaches, and reinforcing the power imbalance by the use of such terminology is unsurprisingly likely to maintain these perceptions. It is helpful to acknowledge the potentially damaging result of the misunderstanding and misapplication of behaviour theory but it is also easy to see how this could occur.

Our final comments centre around the use of the word "holistic" to describe CBA. Despite claiming to be a theory of everything, the physical aspect of Molly's experience has largely been ignored in this formulation, or dismissed as a 'response'. However, as we discussed within our chapter, physiological experience (e.g., IBS, pelvic pain, butterflies, etc.) is an important part of Molly's presentation, as are the 'past traumas' which Molly alludes to being unable to move on from. It seems that these aspects of her experience would be largely ignored amongst the goal-focused behavioural work, potentially dismissing aspects of Molly's experience which make up the 'whole'. Therefore it is doubtful whether CBA can truly be described as holistic, as the whole of the client is not embraced in therapy; rather, aspects of their experience are rejected when they don't fit with the theory.

David M Gresswell, David L Dawson & Nima G Moghaddam

3.7 Author Response

As behaviourists, although we would argue that CBA is not a "*conceptually* reductive system of thought", we do not find the allegation particularly aversive. The use of phrases such as "trust, rapport, collaboration, or empathy" when talking about relationships is of course perfectly reasonable, but as scientists, we want to explore these constructs in more depth, and this deeper level of analysis requires a different, more precise form of understanding and language – language such as that used (and critiqued) in our chapter. When we understand the mechanisms that underpin constructs such as 'collaboration', 'trust', 'rapport', etc., we can identify how to facilitate these more effectively. It is of course important that the client feels safe and contained within the therapeutic vehicle – but if that vehicle breaks down, we need to understand the underlying mechanics and components so that we can get the vehicle running and back on the road again.

As CBA practitioners, we aim to be explicit and transparent about potential power imbalances, negotiating measurable goals in therapy, using methods of intervention that have been empirically derived and tested, and evaluating our effectiveness as therapists – we do not fear exposure or obscure the mechanisms of our practice through the use of vagaries. By contrast, our BCP critics look to achieve goals "that are difficult to put into words".

It is true that, by and large, we take the view "all other approaches are really just crypto-CBA". Radical behaviourism is indeed a theory that accounts for all of human behaviour – including the bodily experiences focused on by our BCP colleagues. This does not mean we cannot learn from other theories, including BCP, although as scientist-practitioners, we are inclined to wait for an evidence-base to develop before taking their concepts on board uncritically.

Finally, behaviourists have sometimes been accused of lacking a sense of humour, but we cannot help but relish the irony of being accused of not "embracing the whole of the client" by "*Body*-Centred Psychotherapists". In fact, for us, the strength of CBA is that it acknowledges that human responses are complex multi-component processes, and that if we want to make credible attempts to understand them, we also need to consider and analyse the contexts that have shaped our responses, and how those contexts elicit and maintain our responses. Our view remains that no other approach is as balanced, explicit, evidence-based, holistic, or transparent in its methods and goals as CBA – consequently we are surprised when our critics attempt to punish our democratic stance. As CBA therapists we find working in this open way reinforcing, and consequently find the prospect of being less collaborative with our clients and not putting our goals "into words", highly aversive.

References

Barlow, D. H., Nock, M., & Hersen, M. (2009). *Single Case Experimental Designs: Strategies for Studying Behavior for Change*. UK: Pearson.

Biglan, A., & Hayes, S. C. (1997). Should the behavioral sciences become more pragmatic? The case for functional contextualism in research on human behavior. *Applied and Preventive Psychology, 5*(1), 47-57.

Brown, F. G., & Gillard, D. (2015). The 'strange death' of radical behaviourism *The Psychologist, 28*(1), 24-27.

Cuijpers, P., van Straten, A., Andersson, G., & van Oppen, P. (2008). Psychotherapy for depression in adults: a meta-analysis of comparative outcome studies. *Journal of Consulting and Clinical Psychology, 76*(6), 909-922.

Cuijpers, P., Van Straten, A., & Warmerdam, L. (2007). Behavioral activation treatments of depression: A meta-analysis. *Clinical Psychology Review, 27*(3), 318-326.

Deacon, B. J., & Abramowitz, J. S. (2004). Cognitive and behavioral treatments for anxiety disorders: a review of meta-analytic findings. *Journal of Clinical Psychology, 60*(4), 429-441.

Eldevik, S., Hastings, R. P., Hughes, J. C., Jahr, E., Eikeseth, S., & Cross, S. (2009). Meta-analysis of early intensive behavioral intervention for children with autism. *Journal of Clinical Child & Adolescent Psychology, 38*(3), 439-450.

Eysenck, H. J. (1968). A theory of the incubation of anxiety/fear responses. *Behaviour Research and Therapy, 6*(3), 309-321.

Fabiano, G. A., Pelham, W. E., Coles, E. K., Gnagy, E. M., Chronis-Tuscano, A., & O'Connor, B. C. (2009). A meta-analysis of behavioral treatments for attention-deficit/hyperactivity disorder. *Clinical Psychology Review, 29*(2), 129-140.

Ferster, C. B. (1973). A functional analysis of depression. *American Psychologist, 28*(10), 857-870.

Feske, U., & Chambless, D. L. (1995). Cognitive behavioral versus exposure only treatment for social phobia: A meta-analysis. *Behavior Therapy, 26*(4), 695-720.

Hageman, W., & Arrindell, W. A. (1999). Establishing clinically significant change: Increment of precision and the distinction between individual and group level of analysis. *Behaviour Research and Therapy, 37*(12), 1169-1193.

Hayes, S. C. (1993). Analytic goals and the varieties of scientific contextualism.

Hayes, S. C., Barnes-Holmes, D., & Roche, B. (2001). *Relational Frame Theory: A post-Skinnerian account of human language and cognition*. New York: Kluwer Academic.

Hayes, S. C., Strosahl, K. D., & Wilson, K. G. (1999). *Acceptance and commitment therapy: An experiential approach to behavior change*: Guilford Press.

Jacobson, N. S., Dobson, K. S., Truax, P. A., Addis, M. E., Koerner, K., Gollan, J. K., . . . Prince, S. E. (1996). A component analysis of cognitive-behavioral treatment for depression. *Journal of Consulting and Clinical Psychology, 64*(2), 295-304.

Jacobson, N. S., Martell, C. R., & Dimidjian, S. (2001). Behavioral activation treatment for depression: Returning to contextual roots. *Clinical Psychology: Science and Practice, 8*(3), 255-270.

Kanter, J. W., Busch, A. M., Weeks, C. E., & Landes, S. J. (2008). The nature of clinical depression: Symptoms, syndromes, and behavior analysis. *The Behavior Analyst, 31*(1), 1-21.

Kazdin, A. E. (2013). *Behavior modification in applied settings* (7th ed.). Long Grove, IL: Waveland Press.

Kobak, K. A., Greist, J. H., Jefferson, J. W., Katzelnick, D. J., & Henk, H. J. (1998). Behavioral versus pharmacological treatments of obsessive compulsive disorder: a meta-analysis. *Psychopharmacology, 136*(3), 205-216.

Kohlenberg, R. J., & Tsai, M. (1991). *Functional Analytic Psychotherapy: Creating Intense and Curative Therapeutic Relationships*. New York: Plenum Press.

Laumann, E. O., Paik, A., Glasser, D. B., Kang, J.-H., Wang, T., Levinson, B., . . . Gingell, C. (2006). A cross-national study of subjective sexual well-being among older women and men: findings from the Global Study of Sexual Attitudes and Behaviors. *Archives of sexual behavior, 35*(2), 143-159.

Laumann, E. O., Paik, A., & Rosen, R. C. (1999). Sexual dysfunction in the United States: prevalence and predictors. *JAMA, 281*(6), 537-544.

Lewinsohn, P. M. (1974). A behavioral approach to depression. In R. M. Friedman & M. M. Katz (Eds.), *The psychology of depression: Contemporary theory and research* (pp. 157-185). New York: Wiley.

Martell, C. R., Addis, M. E., & Jacobson, N. S. (2001). *Depression in context: Strategies for guided action*. New York: WW Norton & Co.

Morley, S. (2013). Single case research. In G. Parry & F. Watts (Eds.), *Behavioural and Mental Health Research: A Handbook of Skills and Methods* (2nd ed., pp. 277-314). UK: Taylor & Francis.

Morley, S., Eccleston, C., & Williams, A. (1999). Systematic review and meta-analysis of randomized controlled trials of cognitive behaviour therapy and behaviour therapy for chronic pain in adults, excluding headache. *Pain, 80*(1), 1-13.

Mowrer, O. (1956). Two-factor learning theory reconsidered, with special reference to secondary reinforcement and the concept of habit. *Psychological Review, 63*(2), 114.

Pavlov, I. P. (1927). *Conditioned Reflexes: An Investigation of the Physiological Activity of the Cerebral Cortex* (G. Anrep, Trans.). Oxford: Oxford University Press.

Pierce, W. D., & Cheney, C. D. (2013). *Behavior analysis and learning*. Hove: Psychology Press.

Skinner, B. F. (1953). *Science and human behavior*. New York: The Free Press.
Skinner, B. F. (1957). *Verbal behavior*. New York: Appleton-Century-Crofts.
Skinner, B. F. (1974). *About behaviorism*. New York: Alfred A. Knopf.
Skinner, B. F. (1989). The origins of cognitive thought. *American Psychologist, 44*(1), 13.
Smith, M. T., Perlis, M. L., Park, A., Smith, M. S., Pennington, J., Giles, D. E., & Buysse, D. J. (2014). Comparative meta-analysis of pharmacotherapy and behavior therapy for persistent insomnia. *American Journal of Psychiatry*.
Thorndike, E. L. (1931). *Human learning*. London: Century.
Watson, J. B. (1919). *Psychology from the standpoint of a behaviorist*. London: J. B. Lippincott & Co.
Weinberger, J., & Rasco, C. (2007). Empirically supported common factors. In S. G. Hofmann & J. Weinberger (Eds.), *The art and science of psychotherapy* (pp. 103-129). New York: Routledge.

Nima G Moghaddam & David L Dawson

4 Cognitive-Behavioural Therapy

In this chapter, the case of Molly is formulated within a cognitive-behavioural therapy (CBT) framework. CBT is a generic term, encompassing both: (1) approaches underpinned by an assumption that presenting emotional and behavioural difficulties are cognitively mediated (A. T. Beck, 2005) or moderated (Hofmann & Asmundson, 2008); and (2) atheoretical bricolages of cognitive and behavioural techniques (Fennell, 1989). This latter category may include *effective* therapeutic packages (perhaps acting through mechanisms articulated in the first category) but, when theory is tacit, it becomes harder to make analytical generalisations or to extrapolate principles that could guide idiographic formulation and intervention. In contrast, the first category of approaches posits that presenting difficulties may be formulated from an assessment of individual cognitive content (thought processes and underlying beliefs) and implies that we can bring about change in presenting difficulties through change in associated cognitions.

Within the expansive category of *theory-linked* CBT approaches, however, there remains a great deal of heterogeneity. Beyond a broadly shared assumption about the influential role of cognitions, we find that variants and developments of CBT place differential emphases on (for example): level of analysis (e.g., situational versus individual); levels of cognition (e.g., immediate thoughts versus underlying core beliefs); problem-specificity (e.g., trans-diagnostic versus disorder-specific); the relative contribution of 'non-cognitive' variables (e.g., overt behaviour, emotional experience, social context); and the particular *mechanism* of cognitive influence (e.g., mediational versus interactional), with some variants hypothesising complex interrelations, involving pathways between multiple cognitive 'systems'. Recent incarnations of CBT seem to place less emphasis on direct cognitive change (i.e., targeting the content, occurrence, and believability of thought processes) and greater emphasis on changing how people attend, relate, and respond to cognitions (i.e., second-order change; Hayes, Villatte, Levin, & Hildebrandt, 2011) – one such model is discussed in Chapter 5 of this volume.

Given the diversity of 'CBT' approaches, and the potentially divergent implications of selecting one model over another, it is important that we specify the particular framework that we will use for the purposes of this chapter. We primarily base our approach and formulation on the theoretical model articulated by A. T. Beck (1976). This model is internally coherent and led to the development of a cohesive system for case formulation (J. S. Beck, 1995; Kuyken, Fothergill, Musa, & Chadwick, 2005). Beck's theory seems to offer a broadly applicable and logical account of functioning, and therapy based specifically on this account has been effective (Knapp & Beck, 2008). Notwithstanding these strengths, we will go on to critique the model, and question some of its fundamental assumptions about mechanism of change and 'active ingredients' of intervention. Nonetheless, we will argue that the theory has a number of strengths that make it a *useful* model (in a pragmatic sense) for the purposes of formulation – particularly in view of the current state of evidence for psychological case conceptualisation.

4.1 Beckian CBT

Beck's CBT model distinguishes between cognition (thoughts, appraisals, and beliefs), emotional experience, and overt behaviour – and emphasises the primacy of cognition: suggesting that our feelings and actions are largely determined by our belief-based appraisals of events (A. T. Beck, 1976; A. T. Beck, Rush, Shaw, & Emery, 1979). A logical implication of this is that when people present with feelings of distress or problematic patterns of behaviour, we can target the way that they think about (appraise) events and other aspects of their life in order to effect therapeutic change. It should be stressed that Beck did not posit cognitions as ultimately causal or aetiological (exogenous) variables, but saw cognitions as a pragmatic point of entry for understanding and intervention. At the point at which a client may present clinically, we do not observe the origins of the problem; rather, we are working with a *cross-section* of current difficulties, which may be informative about proximate influences and maintaining factors without affording insight into ultimate or distal causes. Beck identified cognitions as the first amenable target within a *logical* sequence of situational responses (cognitions, emotions, and behaviours) that reflect and perpetuate presenting difficulties. This *logical* sequence supports practicable understanding of difficulties, although evidence for affective primacy and automaticity (Rachman, 1981; Storbeck & Clore, 2007) suggests that the *actual* sequence of responses to a given situation may be different, and difficult to discern. In essence, the disaggregation of cognitions, emotions, and behaviours into discrete analytical units is largely pragmatic rather than ontological.

As might be expected from the foregoing discussion, CBT treatment focuses on 'here and now' problems and the factors that maintain them; but, importantly, current difficulties are also typically understood to reflect broader, enduring belief systems with origins in earlier experiences. Beck's model posits that developmental experiences produce core beliefs, with contingent beliefs and assumptions that are compensated for by various behavioural and cognitive strategies. Crucially, even where developmental experiences are considered *negative* (e.g., being abused by others), and are seen to produce potentially *maladaptive* core beliefs and secondary assumptions (e.g., others cannot be trusted; to get by, I must depend on myself), we may not see any 'problem' as long as compensatory strategies (e.g., self-reliance, avoidance of others) are working. Difficulties are expected to emerge when *critical incidents* (stressful events or contexts) occur that 'activate' the maladaptive belief system, but also negate the effectiveness of previously engaged compensatory strategies; in our parenthetical example above, this might be because the individual is forced into a position of dependence on others (e.g., due to a deterioration in health). Theoretically, once activated, maladaptive beliefs produce negative thoughts and appraisals – often inferences about a current situation, but also cued expectations about the future or remembrances of the past – with negative emotional and behavioural sequelae. Within the model, maladaptive beliefs are purported to *bias* attention and interpretations (e.g., selective focus on information that 'confirms' negative beliefs about others; discounting of contradictory information) and thus become somewhat self-sustaining and resistant to change.

The simplicity of the model belies its explanatory and therapeutic potential. The notion that people's experiences are shaped by idiographic and enduring beliefs allows us to account for differences between individuals (i.e., why two people may appraise and respond to a similar situation in starkly different ways) and consistencies within individuals (i.e., why a person may act in similar ways across different contexts and occasions). Furthermore, this notion highlights the possibility of achieving lasting, cross-situational changes if we can modify implicated beliefs.

Although Beck's model implies that we should target beliefs directly, it also supports the use of emotion-focussed or behavioural techniques to facilitate cognitive change. For example, preliminary work around emotional tolerance may be needed to enable engagement with cognitive techniques; and behavioural experiments – which proffer the opportunity for direct environmental feedback – may provide the most convincing evidence against irrational and maladaptive thoughts. Within Beck's CBT model, we would expect the most enduring change to arise from shifts in beliefs and thinking patterns, but these shifts may be contingent on changes in emotional or behavioural experiences.

4.2 Historical Origins

Beck's seminal theory was primarily developed on the basis of clinical observations of depression, rather than from research evidence (A. T. Beck, 1976); and knowledge of this development may help us to understand both strengths and weaknesses of the model. The face validity and clinical practicability of CBT would seem to follow from its basis in clinical experience; conversely, there are limitations in the research bases for CBT – in particular, a lack of evidence in support of the central theorised mechanism (cognitive mediation) and separation from broader developments in cognitive science – which likely reflect the fact that research endeavours have been secondary to clinical insight and effectiveness. Empirical studies have provided support for some aspects of Beck's theory (e.g., identifying the presence of expected cognitive themes and biases in particular presentations; A. T. Beck, 2005), but further work is needed to test assumptions regarding the underlying model of change (discussed later).

In terms of wider influences, Beck drew on the proximal work of other cognitive theorists (including Albert Ellis and George Kelly), and was inspired by a (then) recent turn within behavioural psychology towards considering intra-organismic variables or private behaviours that might mediate or moderate responses to the environment (A. T. Beck, 2005; A. T. Beck et al., 1979). Philosophically, Beck linked the tenets of CBT to phenomenological interests in subjective experience and traced them back, for example, to the writings of Greek Stoic philosophers, such as Epictetus and (later) Marcus Aurelius, who observed that people (1) are disturbed by their judgements of events, rather than the events themselves, and (2) have the power to change these judgments and their responses to the events that befall them. Indeed, as Robertson (2010) has observed, the original Stoic writings have a practically instructive and therapeutic focus, which would readily fit with CBT and other modern psychotherapies (such as ACT; Chapter 5).

Beck led a shift away from a focus on behaviour change, which had characterised foregoing behavioural therapies, towards a focus on cognitive change (Hayes et al., 2011). Subsequent years have seen the emergence of a range of cognitive theories and therapies – some of which explicitly draw and develop upon Beck's model (Persons, 2008).

We choose to ground our approach to CBT in Beck's seminal cognitive therapy, and have focussed our account of historical origins accordingly. However, it should be acknowledged that the origins of CBT can be linked to the work of other theorists, and traced back empirically to foundational work in behavioural psychology (see Hawton, Salkovskis, Kirk, & Clark, 1989, for an informative overview). Moreover, CBT can be seen to have been conceptually and practically prefigured by 'rational' approaches to psychotherapy in the early twentieth century (which also took inspiration from Stoic philosophy; Robertson, 2010).

4.3 Defining Features

Both the theory and practice of CBT are typified by a focus on cognition (Longmore & Worrell, 2007). In a review of psychotherapy practices, Blagys and Hilsenroth (2002) identified that CBT treatment activities were distinctively characterised by efforts to identify and change problematic thinking. Other distinguishing features of CBT included: (1) provision of information about the treatment rationale and presenting difficulties (psychoeducation); (2) an emphasis on structured and methodical session activity; (3) an onus on the client completing tasks outside of sessions ('homework'); and (4) development of coping skills to support functioning, both now and in the future (Blagys & Hilsenroth, 2002). Taken together, these features seem consistent with early distinctions made by A. T. Beck et al. (1979), who identified CBT in terms of collaborative empiricism, working with mental processes, and orientating towards current and future experience. For example, the principle of collaborative empiricism

– working with the client to rationally and systematically investigate current difficulties – is evinced in the open sharing of information and psychoeducation, a structured and methodical approach to session activity, and the client's role in collecting evidence outside of sessions.

Notwithstanding the above, we should acknowledge here again that the proliferation of CBT approaches has resulted in diversity, such that it has become difficult to isolate defining features (Hayes et al., 2011) or to critique 'CBT' as a single, coherent approach. One symptom of this is the recent publication of a Delphi study (Morrison & Barratt, 2010) aiming to identify a consensual view of core CBT components (for a single treatment target). The identified need for consensus-building is indicative of the multiplicity of approaches and understandings that are collectively categorised as 'CBT'. Moreover, the study's reliance on practitioner agreement tells us something about the state of evidence for 'active ingredients' in CBT: If we had strong evidence that particular components were associated with therapeutic outcomes (efficacy), the need for a consensus-based method would be largely negated.

4.4 Empirical Evidence

The efficacy of CBT has been the subject of extensive investigation: A recent comprehensive review identified 269 meta-analytic studies of CBT (Hofmann, Asnaani, Vonk, Sawyer, & Fang, 2012) encompassing a broad range of clinical presentations and populations. The review attested to a generally strong evidence-base for efficacy, but this summative conclusion is subject to various qualifications when disaggregated (i.e., specific applications of CBT differ in observed effect sizes or quality of evidence) and there are notable difficulties in pooling findings across a literature of such breadth and heterogeneity.

Further to variability in presentation and population, the magnitude of effects vary according to comparison condition – i.e., whether comparisons were treatment-treatment or treatment-control, and whether controls were passive (e.g., waiting list) or active (e.g., treatment-as-usual) – and these were multifarious. Similarly, evidence was stronger for some presentations (e.g., anxiety disorders) than others (e.g., distress related to medical conditions).

We might be more confident in our ability to integrate the CBT evidence-base if we are assured that, at minimum, there is theoretical consistency across intervention studies – i.e., that we are accumulating evidence for the same *model* of therapeutic change (irrespective of superficial differences in techniques used to deliver, measure, or analyse the hypothesised processes of interest, or in the targeted problems or client groups). However, the heterogeneity of approaches categorised as CBT (beyond basic assumptions) makes it difficult to interpret such evidence as supportive of a singular and distinctive model (i.e., Beck's seminal theory).

4.5 Critique

Strikingly, there is (currently) limited evidence to suggest that findings favouring CBT efficacy are accounted for by putative mechanisms of change. In a comprehensive review of component studies, Longmore and Worrell (2007) identified a lack of empirical support for the central CBT assumption of cognitive primacy. Specifically, studies to date suggest that (1) cognitively-focussed strategies may not contribute to effectiveness over and above behavioural components of CBT (e.g., behavioural activation in depression; Jacobson et al., 1996) and (2) there is little evidence that therapeutic effects of CBT are mediated by cognitive changes. We might expect cognitive change to *accompany* broader therapeutic change, to the extent that cognitions are interdependent with other (e.g., behavioural and emotional) outcomes of interest (e.g., Persons, 2008). However, even if we assume interdependence (an assumption challenged by evidence for desynchrony between cognitive, emotional, and behavioural responses; Rachman, 1981) this broader conceptualisation potentially relegates cognitive change to an epiphenomenal (versus *influential*) role (see Chapter 3).

In practice, component and mediational research may be limited by, for example: (1) the extent to which important cognitive changes are measurable (e.g., accessible to self-report) and the quality of available measures (Jacobson et al., 1996); (2) the extent to which cognitive changes are separable from other changes; and (3) the extent to which CBT can be dismantled into separate components (e.g., purely cognitive versus behavioural strategies) without losing important synergies of the 'whole' approach.

Caveats aside, the recurrent finding of equivalence between various intervention-strategies – within CBT (Longmore & Worrell, 2007) and across psychotherapies more broadly (e.g., Ahn & Wampold, 2001) – may be taken to support the argument that clinical improvements are chiefly accounted for by 'common factors'. If we proceed with this in mind, we may still consider CBT formulation *useful* in so far as it provides a plausible basis for the development of these non-specific components – i.e., formulation may support improvements through facilitation of (for example): client expectancy, therapist confidence and perceived self-efficacy, and an alliance built on shared understanding and goals. At minimum, it would seem important for there to be a clear and credible rationale for engagement in the tasks of therapy, and we would argue that CBT formulation may have particular (potential) strengths here in terms of comprehensibility, simplicity, and face validity.

Our suggestion above is that, in the context of limited evidence for mechanisms hypothesised by the CBT model, the case for *formulating* on the basis of this model may depend on more pragmatic and consequentialist arguments. However, there is a surprising paucity of empirical research examining whether the process of formulation relates to outcomes in CBT. Here again research is limited by complications in measurement and design. It is likely difficult to capture the relationship between formulation and outcome whilst accounting for the myriad variables that may be implicated in intermediary or confounding roles. Efforts to implement more controlled designs have restricted some of the dynamics of formulation in practice (e.g., collaborative development over time, hypothesis testing and reformulation in response to refutational feedback, etc.; Kuyken, Padesky, & Dudley, 2008) and may consequently afford restricted understanding.

4.6 Formulation in Action

Working within the Beckian CBT framework, our approach to formulation is guided by the basic logic of cognitive mediation. At the *situational* level, this suggests that we can understand emotional and behavioural responses to a given event by identifying the individual's thoughts about the event, and inferring its personal meaning (in terms of the individual's underlying assumptions and beliefs). Thus, we might start by identifying an emotionally salient incident for Molly (beginning with either the emotion or the eliciting situation) and then seek to understand the emotional salience of that situation (i.e., bridge from situation to response) by identifying the interceding thoughts and associated ('activated') beliefs. We would normally accomplish this through discussion with Molly, using inference chaining to move from initial thoughts about the situation to underlying meanings and more fundamental beliefs: Here, we are looking to identify beliefs commensurate in content and power to the form and intensity of the emotional responses displayed or reported by the client, and would continue to 'ladder down' until we see a 'good fit' between cognitive and emotional components. This process (in itself) should help to engage Molly with the tenets of the model. For example, by encouraging Molly to discriminate inferences and evaluations about an event from the event itself; and to consider how her responses to a situation reflect her particular interpretations, with the implication that a shift in perspective might lead her to feel and act differently. To foster recognition of this latter implication, we may begin to explore how different interpretations of the same event might have produced quite different reactions. Interactive formulation and guided discovery around implications of the model are consistent with the core CBT principle of collaborative empiricism: intended to inculcate client ownership and self-efficacy, and thereby potentiate other processes of therapy (although the model-specific rationale for this 'motivational' component is not well-specified; Ryan, Lynch, Vansteenkiste, & Deci, 2011).

A parallel process occurs at the *developmental* level. Again, we are attempting to explain a process in terms of interceding cognitive variables; in this case, we wish to understand how an individual's current problems might be linked to earlier experiences, in terms of the particular beliefs that have been formed from these experiences. In cases where there is a clear 'critical incident' leading to referral, we would seek to comprehend the 'critical' nature of the precipitating incident through our developmental understanding of the beliefs that it may have activated: We would expect to find that the critical incident is analogous, in terms of *meaning*, to earlier belief-formative experiences. We would normally identify implicated core beliefs at the situational level of formulation (as described above); clients may find it difficult to report on core beliefs (Lemmens et al., 2014) and situational analyses may enable collaborative discovery of these by grounding the inferential process in data from specific experiences. However, it is possible (and sometimes necessary, as here) to identify recurrent patterns of thinking in clients' accounts of their broader history and general in-session talk. We might begin to infer beliefs on this basis, later checking inferences for resonance with clients, and testing for triangulation in subsequent situational analyses.

In Molly's case, we are unable to build our formulation directly with her, and the following initial formulation is predicated on the material available in Chapter 2. With limited situational detail to draw upon, and given the historical narrative of Molly's case, we place greater emphasis here on the developmental aspect of formulation. We use Judith Beck's (1995) case conceptualisation diagram for developmental formulation as it provides a clear, understandable account of case presentations (Kuyken et al., 2005) based on the Beckian model. Molly's beliefs and strategies are inferred from the documented developmental history and analysis of described problem situations/critical events, with attention to Molly's own words where available. At the situational level, our approach to formulation is adapted from Ellis' ABC (Activating event, Beliefs, Consequences) model (Chadwick, Birchwood, & Trower, 1996; Ellis, 2004). Working within the CBT model, we are sensitive to our own susceptibility to bias and how this may influence formulation: Through a collaborative empirical approach, we would remain open to disconfirmation of initial hypotheses and revisit/revise formulation in response to on-going information-gathering.

A question that arises when applying CBT formulation with a particular case is whether to use a problem-specific model. It may be possible to identify that the client presents with a particular clinical problem or 'disorder' (e.g., depression) and select a template approach that is specific to that problem/disorder. Such templates typically adapt the generic Beckian model to identify problem-specific cognitive profiles and other characteristics. Problem-specific models have been used to develop manualised CBT treatments, which have demonstrated efficacy (Dudley, Kuyken, & Padesky, 2011), and some have argued that the most defensible approach to case formulation is to apply a problem-specific template (Grant, Townend, Mills, & Cockx, 2008) – if one is available and has been used in an empirically-supported treatment protocol. Against this, as discussed above, we lack evidence that treatments work *because* of their problem-specific components, or that template-based formulations contribute to efficacy. As clinicians, we also consider it problematic to make assumptions based on topography (apparently similar presentations may have divergent causes/underlying cognitions) and 'fitting' clients to prototypic formulations may lose the potentially idiographic and cross-diagnostic strengths of the broader model (and potentially undermine 'collaborative' principles). Moreover, in practice we commonly see mixed presentations that may be ill-served by a problem-specific framework.

4.6.1 Initial Formulation

4.6.1.1 Early Life

Theoretically, early experiences shape core beliefs that may be activated by analogous experiences in later life (A. T. Beck et al., 1979); thus, examination of childhood and other historical data may facilitate a developmental understanding of current problems.

Molly described her home life as lacking 'warmth': She experienced her parents as distant (from her and from each other) yet controlling, and strived to attain their affection (reduce this distance) by meeting perceived demands (e.g., in terms of attainment and self-reliance). However, Molly's salient recollections are of times when she seemed to fall short of (her mother's) standards and a sense of being unfavourably compared to her sister Ella. Of particular significance for Molly's development, we would hypothesise, was learning that emotions should not be expressed or dealt with directly. Molly's parents were seemingly critical and invalidating of her feelings (conveying that she was "overly emotional" and "dramatic") and modelled emotional avoidance in their own behaviour. Further to suppression of negative emotions, there is a notable absence of *positive* emotion in Molly's account of her early life.

Compounding learning from home, Molly experiences difficulties in forming/maintaining relationships at school, and again understands this as a rejection of her "emotionally demanding" behaviour.

Molly's experience of sexual abuse may have influenced conceptions of self (as vulnerable and shameful/"dirty") and others (threatening/untrustworthy; e.g., Rieckert & Möller, 2000). Her tacit, isolative response to the abuse likely reflects early familial emphases on self-reliance and emotional inhibition/non-confrontation – and may have contributed to the formation of compensatory strategies that would later prove problematic (e.g., attempts to control, escape, or avoid emotions). However, we would be cautious about over-interpreting the role of the abuse experience at this stage: There is considerable correlational evidence for links between childhood abuse, dysfunctional cognitive development, and psychological difficulties in adulthood (Trickett & McBride-Chang, 1995), but a cognition-predicated formulation should place abuse (and any other potentially salient experience) within a broader (idiographic) developmental perspective, and prioritise the personal meaning/implications of the experience for the client, rather than the a priori assumptions of the therapist.

4.6.1.2 Core Beliefs

It is possible to infer fundamental beliefs emergent from Molly's early life experiences.

My feelings are unacceptable and dangerous. Such a belief may develop from Molly's early experiences of expressed feelings being invalidated (chiefly by her parents) and the perceived isolative consequences of being "overly emotional" (i.e., the impression that others withdrew from her because she was too "emotionally demanding"). The notion of feelings as dangerous may have subsequently been strengthened by adult experiences of coping difficulties – e.g., Molly's overdose and self-cutting may have been attempts to escape from overwhelming feelings of distress. This inferred belief reflects cognitive themes of both responsibility (there is something in me that is 'faulty') and vulnerability (sharing my feelings and showing my 'faults' is unsafe).

I am "weak and useless". Molly's early experiences may have contributed to self-perceptions of vulnerability and ineffectualness, reflected in Molly's description of herself as "weak and useless". Molly perceived that she was expected (by her mother) to do well without support (i.e., to function with high self-efficacy); thus, any difficulties/failures experienced may have been interpreted by Molly as personal weakness (here, weakness includes a sense of the self as lacking competence or, in Molly's words, "useless"). Molly's perceived inability to control her emotions may also support a belief in the self as weak. In this way, failure to compensate for one belief (unacceptability of emotions) may have strengthened the development of another belief (I am weak and vulnerable to my emotions). Molly's experience of being abused may have further contributed to a belief in the self as weak/vulnerable to exploitation by others.

I don't deserve love. Molly described her childhood home as lacking "warmth" and had a strong sense that she was less loved than her sister. Evidence suggests that children are less able to modify/correct egocentric interpretations of experiences than adults (Epley, Morewedge, & Keysar, 2004). It follows that Molly may have taken personal responsibility for her parents' cold distancing: parsing these experiences as indicative of the self as undeserving of love or affection. Molly's difficulties in forming friendships at school may have served to strengthen the development of this belief.

Others are critical, rejecting, and unsafe. Molly perceived her parents to be critical and rejecting (a perception recurrent in other close relationships with friends and partners) and alleges sexual abuse: The people she depended on hurt her/failed to protect her as a child, and this may have shaped a view of the world/others as cruel and unsafe – closely linked to a belief in the self as vulnerable.

4.6.1.3 Conditional Assumptions

Theoretically, conditional assumptions may facilitate coping with painful core beliefs, but the rules and compensatory strategies that they prompt often prove maladaptive (J. S. Beck, 1995). A number of conditional assumptions (or subsidiary beliefs) may arise from the core beliefs posited for Molly; some possible conditional assumptions are described below:

If I depend on myself, I won't be able to cope AND If I depend on others, then I will be taken advantage of and/or abandoned. The putative core beliefs held by Molly may produce conflicting assumptions around dependency/relating to others. A belief in the self as weak/useless may undermine self-efficacy and suggest the need to rely on others. However, Molly has other beliefs – others are dangerous and she is unlovable – suggesting that she cannot afford to trust or depend on others (given her inherent vulnerability): people will take advantage of her (they are unsafe) and/or they will eventually reject her (she is undeserving of love). Another assumption relating to a belief in the self as weak/incompetent is:

If I cannot function alone, then I am weak and useless. Molly learned from her mother that she should succeed independently, such that struggles and failures may be assumed to confirm perceived weakness.

If I express/have emotions, I am weak. Given a belief in emotions as unacceptable, failure to suppress/avoid emotions (i.e., to uphold personal rules) may be interpreted as personal weakness, and strengthen the core belief 'I am weak'. More simply, each emotional episode appears to confirm beliefs that emotions are dangerous (uncontrollable) and that Molly is vulnerable.

If I feel strong emotions, then I must do something to get rid of them. Such an assumption derives directly from a belief in the unacceptability and dangerousness of feelings (and prior learning, from her parents, that emotions are unacceptable). This assumption might be implicated in Molly's overdose and self-cutting behaviours, which could be understood to function as attempts to escape overwhelming feelings of distress.

If I cannot meet others' standards, then I don't deserve love. A core belief in the self as undeserving of affection may establish and augment monitoring of acceptability to others, with each perceived slight or rejection processed as confirmatory evidence for this belief. Potentially, such a conditional principle could support self-worth: If Molly perceived that she was meeting others' standards she might challenge the core belief that she does not deserve love. In reality, the condition is too stringent (and Molly's other rules and beliefs likely bias her perceptions of attainment and what is expected of her), such that the core belief will be strengthened – and Molly may become increasingly vigilant/frantic in efforts to gauge and modulate her relationships with others.

4.6.1.4 Compensatory Strategies, Presentation, and Maintenance

Molly appears to use various cognitive and behavioural strategies to manage stressors that relate to, or activate, her beliefs. These strategies may have served to trigger her presenting problems and represent important maintaining factors for her distress (preventing disconfirmation of dysfunctional beliefs). The cumulative ineffectiveness of these strategies may contribute to a general sense of hopelessness (supporting Molly's depressive presentation) and related tension.

Attempts to control, avoid, or escape emotions. Molly uses a number of extreme strategies to manage her emotions (Coggins & Fox, 2009). These strategies likely developed in response to a core belief that emotions are endangering and unacceptable, and subsidiary beliefs that showing emotion is a weakness and feelings cannot be tolerated.

Molly attempts to control or inhibit her emotions; however, this strategy may have paradoxical outcomes (rebound effects) and ultimately reinforce Molly's belief that her emotions are dangerous and unacceptable. Molly likely finds that her emotions 'build' – efforts to suppress emotions and associated thoughts may ironically increase salience/preoccupation and amplify emotional intensity – and (eventually) overwhelm her control. When emotions surface after suppression, they tend to be expressed explosively (as observed within the first therapy session) – alarming and embarrassing Molly, and provoking negative reactions in those who experience her outbursts (evident in accounts of Molly as "histrionic", "overly emotional", and "attention-seeking"). The apparent unpredictability of such expressions and the interpersonal difficulties they generate motivates Molly to try harder to control her emotions, increasing her frustration and maintaining the cycle. Molly attempted to use emotional control strategies as a child, learning that emotional expression at home would not be tolerated. Although the strategy may have temporarily helped her to cope in that context (and was an understandable response to invalidation and apparent abuse), it meant that Molly did not learn how to safely experience and express emotion. From early experiences (e.g., at school) to now, this strategy of over-control appears to contribute to interpersonal difficulties and unstable relationships – a presenting issue of concern for Molly.

Molly may also compensate for her beliefs around emotion in an avoidant manner. We see this, for example, in her tendency to evade communication with others when this may involve contact with difficult feelings or emotional confrontation. Relatedly, recently developed habits (e.g., cleaning, TV watching, and snacking) may also function to avoid and distract from emotional experiences. We would be interested in exploring Molly's help-seeking for medical complaints and wonder whether this has been compensatory: Enabling Molly to attain *some* support whilst avoiding implications of acknowledging emotional needs.

Molly's overdose may also be understandable as an attempt to escape from emotional pain; similarly, her self-cutting behaviour whilst in hospital may have enabled respite from contact with distress (by changing her interoceptive focus to physical pain). Recent fasting behaviour could serve an analogue function, in that physical discomfort replaces psychological discomfort, but may also be understandable as a means of attaining perceived standards of others (Molly seems to consider herself too "frumpy" to deserve a partner).

Attempts to control, avoid, and escape emotions should therefore be understood as a linked repertoire of compensatory strategies for emotional regulation. Unfortunately, the self-invalidating nature of this repertoire functions to increase her emotional dysregulation, making it harder for Molly to recognise/track her feelings and modulate her behavioural responses to them.

Depending on others/Mistrust and isolation. Molly uses conflicting strategies in relating to others: she is dependent on others but also mistrusts them. These strategies likely developed in response to beliefs around personal weakness/incompetence (dependence) and others as unsafe and rejecting (mistrust; augmented by intermediate rules and assumptions about the value of self-reliance and being "able to get on with things").

Being dependent on others is understandable as a strategy to compensate for perceived vulnerability, but also limits the ability of an individual to develop personal strength or self-efficacy (i.e., challenge personal perceptions of weakness). This might not be too damaging if Molly could consistently rely on others to protect her, but the dependent strategy is undermined by another strategy: mistrust and isolation. Again, this may have been functional in protecting against perceived external dangers (established by early experiences of criticism, rejection, and abuse – in a context where caregivers were "not really there" for her), but it undermines the possibility of developing genuine reciprocal relationships. Molly's relationships are destabilised by the push and pull of contradictory compensatory strategies: We can see how strategies adopted to aid coping have broken down and may now contribute to/ perpetuate presenting difficulties.

Vigilance for, and efforts to avoid, rejection. In response to perceived threats (others as unsafe), and a sense of self as weak and unlovable, Molly seems to be hyper-vigilant for signs of danger. This strategy closely relates to mistrusting others and is, again, understandable in the context of Molly's early experiences and emergent beliefs. However, the negative expectations that drive this strategy are likely to become self-fulfilling: Either because Molly is overly sensitive in her interpretations – finding 'proof' of her beliefs in ambiguous experiences – or because her guarded/ withdrawn behaviour provokes negative responses in others ('confirming' her concerns – a pattern observed in her experiences at university and as a classroom assistant). Molly expects to be rejected (undeserving), and is sensitive to any cue that she is not fully acceptable to others – often withdrawing pre-emptively in a manner that prevents disconfirmation. It is possible to see that Molly's threat-focused strategy/ bias feeds itself and ultimately isolates her from others, with likely consequences for reinforcing negative core beliefs and the manifestation of anxiety and depression.

Further to pre-emptive withdrawal, Molly sometimes strives to avoid rejection through efforts to appease others (a strategy evident from childhood) – compensating for notions of the self as undeserving of affection, and others as critical and rejecting, by attempting to meet perceived conditions for affection. It is notable that many of her concerns and goals are expressed in other-directed terms – she worries that she has "let everyone down" and wants to "make everyone proud" – and that she subjugates her own suffering (experiences of abuse and hospitalisation) to concerns that she will "wreck the family". Currently, Molly performs errands and chores for her parents in an apparent attempt to atone for her 'failure' to uphold their expected standards.

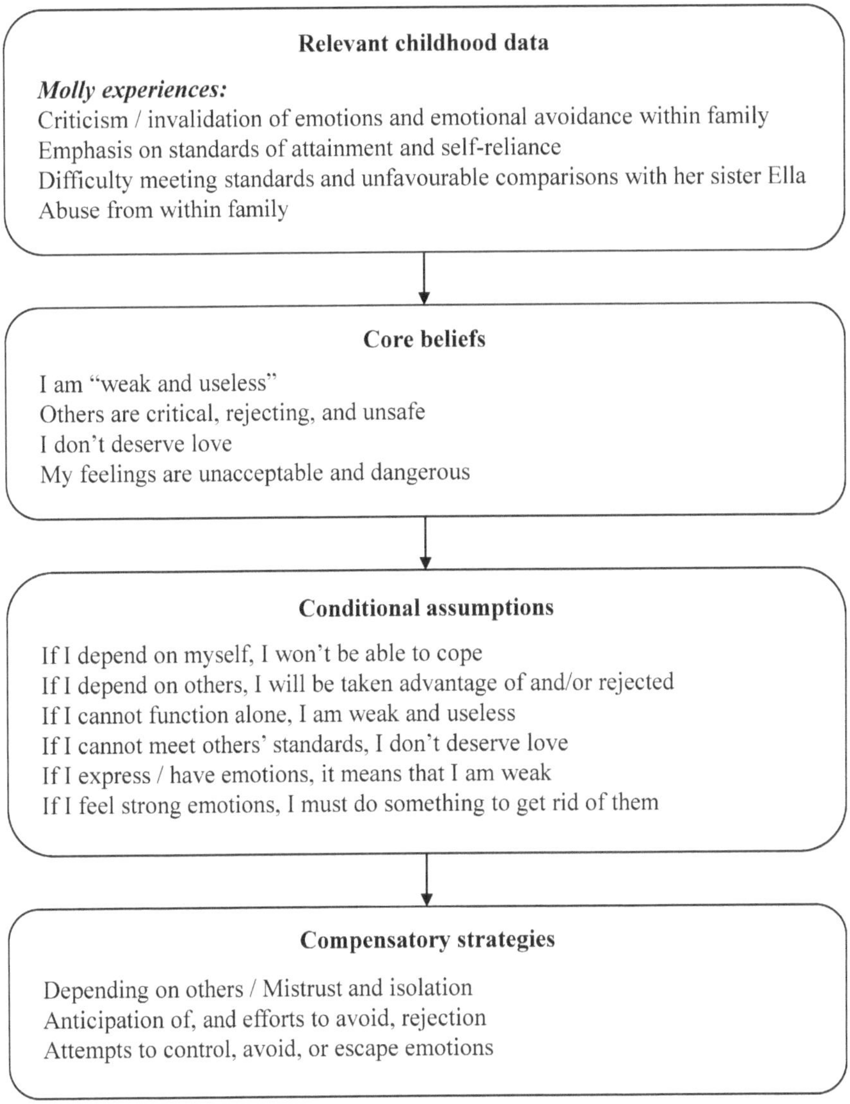

Figure 4.1: Developmental CBT formulation

4.6.2 Situational Formulation

It should be possible to analyse a number of situations in Molly's current/recent experience and find evidence of the maintaining factors and underlying beliefs responsible for her on-going distress. One specific situation is examined here, on the basis of information available.

As previously stated, situational formulation follows a basic ABC structure (Chadwick et al., 1996), with consequences explicitly sub-divided into emotions and behavioural/other outcomes (so as to foster the client's ability to discriminate these, functionally related but discrete, sequelae; Trower, Jones, Dryden, & Casey, 2011). To make the distinction clear, we implement an extended **ABCO** sequence: Specifying the **A**ctivating event, **B**eliefs (about A), emotional **C**onsequences (of B), and ensuing behavioural or other **O**utcomes.

A recent critical incident for Molly is the event that precipitated her withdrawal from Amy and her work colleagues – analogous to earlier relationship patterns (shifting from dependence to avoidance). Figure 4.2 presents an ABCO analysis of this incident.

Activating event	Beliefs (thoughts and images about 'A')	Emotional Consequence of 'B'	Behavioural or other Outcomes
Distant laughter and conversation between friend (Amy) and another colleague	*Inferences* They are laughing at me They don't really like me *Evaluation* I am not acceptable I cannot trust others *Core beliefs (activated)* I don't deserve love Others are critical, rejecting, and unsafe	Shame Anxiety	Withdrawal (protective but isolative) Increased opportunity for rumination (rehearsing and strengthening beliefs) Decreased opportunity for disconfirmation of beliefs

Figure 4.2: Situational ABCO formulation

Within the cognitive model, problematic consequences (shame and isolative withdrawal) are seen to arise from beliefs about the activating event rather than the event itself. In this case (A), Molly's interpretation that her colleagues are ridiculing her (B) evokes shame (C), and motivates withdrawal (O) as a protective response. It's not clear that Molly's interpretation of the distant conversation and laughter is accurate; it may reflect a personalisation or self-referential bias – relating external events to the self without basis (A. T. Beck et al., 1979) – potentiated by vigilance for rejection. Whether accurate or not, Molly's subsequent behaviour suggests overgeneralisation from this incident to conclude that her colleagues don't really like her (regardless of her heretofore close relationship with Amy and other colleagues). Her evaluations are likely to be totalising negative judgements of herself and others, rather than appraisals of the specific experience.In Figure 4.2, we contend that feelings of shame and anxiety could arise from appraisals of the same situation. However, we would help Molly to see these as different emotions associated with different beliefs: Shame pertains to the perceived exposure of personal inadequacy (self as undeserving/"an embarrassment"), whereas anxiety relates to the impression that others are colluding against her (i.e., interpersonal threat/vulnerability – others as critical, rejecting, and unsafe). It may be preferable to present these as separate sequences for Molly: Indeed, we would generally limit the use of formulations that list multiple problem emotions (Cs) as these are generally not helpful in *discriminating* emotional experiences, or making logical sense of how different emotions might arise (i.e., understanding consistency between B-C connections).

Although withdrawal is protective in the short-term, it leaves Molly isolated and thereby reinforces her negative beliefs about self and others. By considering the repercussions of her response to the situation (under O) we can see how Moly's problems may perpetuate – for example, withdrawal reduces opportunities to contact external events (e.g., positive feedback from colleagues) that might disconfirm negative thoughts arising from this incident and provide experiential evidence against broader beliefs.

4.6.3 Intervention Objectives and Evaluation

Intervention would be directed towards Molly's goals, but these are currently quite vague and (as discussed above) framed in terms of others' needs – we would wish to explore these further as stated goals may reflect, among other phenomena, conditional beliefs about meeting others' standards. We expect that collaborative goal-setting may be initially difficult (given Molly's history of subjugating personal needs) and may need to be revisited and revised as therapy proceeds and changes open up different ways of thinking about herself, others, and her future. To enable us to specify and prioritise Molly's presenting concerns, and monitor progress towards addressing these concerns (in a manner consistent with our collaboratively empirical approach), we might use an idiographic weekly measure like the Simplified Personal Questionnaire (Elliott, 2002).

Further to idiographic monitoring and on-going qualitative feedback, we would likely use validated outcome scales pertaining to presenting difficulties (e.g., measures of emotional distress – providing that these captured outcomes relevant to Molly). An advantage of implementing such measures is that we can then use reference data on measurement reliability and population norms to evaluate the statistical reliability and 'clinical significance' of any changes that Molly reports over the course of therapy (i.e., whether changes are beyond what could be attributable to chance or measurement error, and whether change constitutes a shift from clinical to normative levels of distress; Jacobson & Truax, 1991).

If we wish to evaluate whether any observed changes are attributable to theorised mechanisms, we need to measure hypothesised mediating variables. Within CBT, we might thus focus on monitoring change in targeted cognitions (e.g., believability of problem beliefs identified in Molly's formulation). By repeatedly measuring both the proposed mediator (belief in targeted cognitions) and outcome (problem severity) over the course of therapy we can potentially evaluate formulated mediational hypotheses by establishing whether: (1) believability is related to problem severity, (2) our intervention changes believability, and (3) changes in believability precede changes in problem severity (Kazdin, 2009; Mumma, 2004).

Notwithstanding the above, we would be cautious about drawing conclusions based on self-report alone; we would be mindful of the *function* of Molly's self-report, and would explore her presentation accordingly. Essentially, Molly's responses may be subject to various biases (e.g., minimising difficulties and over-reporting therapy benefits, in accordance with a tendency to please others – or maximising difficulties, to avoid termination of therapy, in accordance with dependent strategies) and we would look for evidence of improved functional outcomes and social validation of change (i.e., triangulation with external observations) where possible.

4.6.4 Intervention Plan

Initial efforts would focus on forming therapeutic engagement – through discussion of expectations of the therapy process, formulation sharing, goal-setting, and intervention planning – interpolating experience-normalising psychoeducation around the CBT model, and establishing a collaborative relationship from the outset.

Central to intervention would be modification of the beliefs implicated in Molly's presenting difficulties. We would agree on initial targets here and might use a range of strategies to facilitate a change in perspective (e.g., Trower et al., 2011):

(1) Verbal methods, including targeted Socratic, leading, and assumptive questioning to engage Molly in generating alternative ways of thinking. For example, we might explore the truth of her absolute (negative) evaluations of self and others in the light of exceptions (e.g., her longstanding relationship with Eve). It is notable that our initial formulation focuses on problems and perhaps neglects areas of extant strength (Kuyken et al., 2008). We think it is important to firstly understand (and validate) the difficulties that Molly has experienced, and expect that Molly would initially be dismissive of a 'strengths-focussed' formulation, but would also want to harness existing assets to enable Molly to dispute problem beliefs – attention to positives, disconfirmations, and exceptions becomes crucial here.

(2) Behavioural methods, encouraging Molly to test targeted beliefs by acting in ways that contradict negative thinking, and assessing the outcomes of this. For example, Molly might be asked to approach situations that could lead to rejection or shaming (e.g., initiating conversation with colleagues), as opportunities to learn

that expected consequences may not occur, or (if they do occur), can be tolerated and do not have to be interpreted as totalising (i.e., having internal, global, and stable implications).

(3) Imagery-based methods, including practicing of alternative thinking to imagined situations. For example, Molly may not find alternative ways of thinking convincing when generated in the abstract, but may find behavioural tests too daunting (at first). Imaginal techniques could help Molly to make vivid contact with problem situations and sequelae, eliciting associated thoughts and feelings 'in the room' (experiential versus intellectual insight), before rehearsing alternative thought processes and observing any change in feelings. Imaginal practice may help to catalyse cognitive methods and prepare engagement in behavioural methods.

Although intervention strategies may be discussed, modelled, and practiced within sessions, CBT places an onus on application outside of therapy such that Molly's learning and alternative ways of thinking generalise beyond the therapy context.

Supplementary to strategies focussed on changing beliefs (i.e., the B in the ABCO sequence above) we may also attempt to modulate the occurrence of activating events (A). In terms of activating events, we expect that Molly's behaviour (e.g., social withdrawal) may increase the occurrence of events (being disregarded or criticised by others) that trigger negative beliefs (self as undeserving, others as rejecting/critical) and consequent distress. A focus here might be the development of behavioural skills for effective emotional expression: Molly has not had opportunity to learn how to communicate her needs directly, and we would hypothesise that this potentiates activating events. Development of skills around emotional communication and asserting personal needs should also help to challenge Molly's beliefs about herself as ineffectual and the unacceptability of emotions.

4.6.4.1 Potential Difficulties

We would need to be considerate of how Molly's beliefs may influence her responses to therapy, and would explicitly tackle her thoughts in relation to the therapy process (with potential for more general impact). In this way, in-therapy problems can become important learning opportunities.

Molly may vacillate between dependence and distancing in her relationship with the therapist and, given previous patterns, there is a risk that she could withdraw from therapy in response to perceived ruptures (she is likely to anticipate abandonment and be vigilant for signs of rejection) or experiences of being "exposed" within therapy (activating beliefs about being undeserving and unacceptable, with concomitant shame and avoidance). Molly's rules around self-reliance might potentiate any impulse to withdraw: She already evinces ambivalence around therapy and hates "being so needy".

CBT would place an onus on Molly to complete inter-sessional tasks and be an active collaborator in therapy: There is potential for this to prompt concerns around self-efficacy and ability to meet others' standards, presenting both opportunities (to expose to and challenge such concerns) and threats (for consolidation of beliefs and disengagement). Given a putative belief around the unacceptability of her own emotions (and related avoidant strategies), our primary concern would be with Molly's ability to engage with and tolerate the *emotional* focus of therapy. It may be important to do some initial work around emotion regulation and distress tolerance: Over time, we might enable Molly to manage her emotions through cognitive reappraisal, but we may initially need to rely on more 'response-focussed' strategies – i.e., changing behavioural outcomes (Os) of emotions when activated, through relaxation or response prevention – which would secondarily help Molly to challenge beliefs around the unacceptability and dangerousness of her feelings.

David M Gresswell

4.7 CBT Formulation: Critical Commentary

The authors offer a succinct review of the principles of CBT, along with a critical overview – stressing, in effect, that a CBT formulation is not a literal formulation of how the client functions, but a way of ordering information that helps the client gain access to their experiences. Although not the fault of Beck, the cognitive model seems to have taken on a life of its own in recent years, and it is not uncommon to see it being used as if it represents a coherent model of human action. In this chapter, the authors make the point that the evidence for the primacy of cognition (a central principle of CBT theory) is weak, and that what is helpful in CBT is the attempt to make sense of how certain events have acquired specific meanings – in specific contexts – and how those meanings affect emotional experience.

The ABCO model used by the authors for "the situational formulation" (Molly observing her colleagues laughing – Fig. 4.2) has the advantage over a conventional ABC approach in that it provides two triangulation points with respect to the internal validity of the formulation. Although the components of an emotional experience (private events, physiology, overt behaviours) are not always synchronised, they should be consistent in an ABCO analysis: the 'B' should match not only the 'C' (the emotion) but also the 'O' (the behavioural or other outcome arising from the emotion) in terms of both content and intensity. If the components do not match – e.g., the 'B' seems more consistent with an angry response than an anxious one, but the 'C' is anxiety and the 'O' involves a range of depressive behaviours – then this may indicate that the formulation should be revisited. Despite its advantages, the ABCO approach compounds the criticism that CBT awards spurious primacy to cognition, by additionally giving primacy to emotion over behaviour. Indeed, in the example given in Figure

4.2, the authors appear to ignore the contextual consequences of Molly's behaviours – clearly, as set out here, this model does not provide a coherent and holistic formulation of Molly's problems that matches with what we know about the reality of human experience.

The authors also make the fundamental mistake of including two emotional experiences (shame and anxiety) in the 'C' column – neither of which is clearly predicted by the 'Bs' that are hypothesised to precede them. The authors have not pursued inference chaining to a logical conclusion: why should "they are laughing at me" be linked to the core belief of "I don't deserve love" or to the behavioural outcome (e.g. withdrawal) specified? The authors have not used the triangulation checks available: best practice in CBT is to follow one emotion at a time (rather than the purported core belief), and to be clear about whether inductive or deductive reasoning is being assumed. However, irrespective of whether inductive or deductive reasoning is assumed, it is not obvious why – if Molly believes she "doesn't deserve love" and that "others are critical, rejecting and unsafe" – she should be prone to interpreting the laughter of others as being directed at her, or to reacting with shame or anxiety rather than with anger or depression. Something is missing from this analysis.

A related critique can also be levied at the developmental formulation described in Figure 4.1. The model follows a linear progression from childhood "data" (a misleading use of the term "data" if ever there was one) leading to the formation of core beliefs, then to the extrapolation of conditional assumptions, and finally to the development of compensatory strategies. In reality, when working with Molly, what we are most likely to see first are the "compensatory strategies", *then* to hear Molly's description of her childhood. In this model, there appears to be a real danger of the core beliefs becoming evidence to support Molly's account of her childhood and vice-versa – this is all very circular and not very testable. We cannot observe Molly's childhood and indeed there is some contrary evidence that her sister came out of virtually the same context psychologically intact.

Nevertheless, given their observations, the authors then set out to fill the gap between Molly's account of her childhood and her current presentation – this endeavour produces some rather incoherent results. For example, if Molly actually fully endorsed the core belief "I don't deserve love" then she could not also assume (conditionally or otherwise) "if I cannot meet others' standards then I don't deserve love". She either deserves love or she does not, and the corollary of this conditional assumption is surely: "if I can meet others' standards then I do deserve love". Indeed, this corollary statement would seem far more consistent with Molly's behaviour and her frustrations than the original statement. A similar critique can be applied to the other core beliefs and conditional assumptions – and, as phrased here, it would seem more likely that the "conditional assumptions" lead to the formation of the "core beliefs" than vice-versa – but perhaps the issue is one of nuance?

In summary, it can be seen that both the approaches to CBT formulation expounded here are flawed – the models offered are internally inconsistent; they lack coherence with both mainstream psychology, human experience, and are largely untestable. The use of the construct "core belief" leads to the production of statements that lack nuance and which appear incompatible with the conditional assumptions they allegedly produce. Finally, and perhaps most fatally, the interaction of the client with the outside world is largely ignored. Indeed, irrespective of what a few ancient Greeks had to say on the subject, some situations are intolerable and thinking about them differently won't fix that – sometimes a little behaviour change is required and, that being the case, we need to pay more attention to context and observable behaviours in our formulations and less to hypothetical private events.

Nima G Moghaddam & David L Dawson

4.8 Author Response

We stated our openness to additional information and feedback, whether corrective of the data or our interpretations. However, we were not convinced that the offered critique had implications for refining our initial hypotheses. The commentary appeared to focus on details taken out of context of the broader formulation (selective abstraction?) and to make some arbitrary inferences that were contrary to available evidence (perhaps more reflective of the commentator's preconceptions about the case material and formulation model?).

Fragmentary reading of the formulation is suggested by the manner in which the 'situational' and 'developmental' aspects of the broader formulation are critiqued separately, without consideration of their inter-connectedness. The commentator states that we have "not used the triangulation checks available", but neglects that the situational and developmental levels of analysis are points of triangulation for each other, providing complementary insights.

For example, the commentator takes issue with the inference chain in Figure 4.2 (questioning how laughter from others might connect to an underlying sense of the self as undeserving) but we would suggest that the linkage here is elaborated at length (and connected to earlier experiences) within the broader formulation and developmental narrative (over-vigilance for rejection, and a conditional belief that rejection from others means she is underserving). Similarly, the commentator appears to read the figures as independent from the broader analytic narrative: the two are interdependent, and the textual description should help to expound links within the (necessarily reductive) figures – just as, in practice, we would not share a diagrammatic formulation without elaborative discussion. For example, within the text accompanying Figure 4.2, we do acknowledge potential confusion that can arise from considering two emotional experiences together – and explicitly discriminate these in terms of their phenomenological correlates.

In challenging our analysis, the commentator appears to draw less on the information available than on expectations about how people 'should' respond in Molly's situation. Returning to Figure 4.2: We might ask *why* Molly did not express anger or confront her colleagues, but the material tells us that she responded with withdrawal and worry, and that such responses are part of a consistent pattern of self-blaming/ tendencies towards shame and wariness of others. Of course, questions of external correspondence remain (and would be examined in therapy with Molly) but we argue that the formulation is grounded in currently available data – and is internally consistent.

Putting aside our own reservations about the utility of core belief constructs[2], the critique here seems to misrepresent their theorised role: To reiterate, negative core beliefs are not consistently active/manifest (or "fully endorsed") and conditional assumptions or rules are developed to protect against their activation. The suggestion that external context is 'largely ignored' also seems misrepresentative: Analysis in CBT encompasses interactions with the outside world but deliberately focusses on how these come to shape and be understood through individual appraisals (Beck, 1976). The commentator's definition of 'context' appears somewhat constricted here – e.g., the suggestion that Molly and her ("psychologically intact") sister emerged from "virtually the same context" seems to ignore salient differences in environmental feedback/relational context.

References

Ahn, H., & Wampold, B. E. (2001). Where oh where are the specific ingredients? A meta-analysis of component studies in counseling and psychotherapy. *Journal of Counseling Psychology, 48*(3), 251-257.

Beck, A. T. (1976). *Cognitive therapy and the emotional disorders.* New York: International Universities Press.

Beck, A. T. (2005). The current state of cognitive therapy: A 40-year retrospective. *Archives of General Psychiatry, 62*(9), 953-959.

Beck, A. T., Rush, A. J., Shaw, B. F., & Emery, G. (1979). *Cognitive therapy of depression: A treatment manual.* New York: Guilford Press.

Beck, J. S. (1995). *Cognitive therapy: Basics and beyond.* New York: Guilford Press.

Blagys, M. D., & Hilsenroth, M. J. (2002). Distinctive activities of cognitive–behavioral therapy: A review of the comparative psychotherapy process literature. *Clinical Psychology Review, 22*(5), 671-706.

2 We do wonder whether inclusion of core belief constructs may 'over fit' the model. For understanding Molly's day-to-day experiences and behaviour, her conditional assumptions and related strategies are likely to be much more informative than constructs that are (by definition) latent and non-specific. Indeed, there is perhaps a danger of losing important information about an individual's experiences – and consequently, about the particular intermediate beliefs and assumptions that the individual might develop – when these experiences are reduced into generic absolute statements (core beliefs).

Chadwick, P., Birchwood, M., & Trower, P. (1996). *Cognitive therapy for delusions, voices and paranoia*. Chichester: Wiley.

Coggins, J., & Fox, J. R. E. (2009). A qualitative exploration of emotional inhibition: A basic emotions and developmental perspective. *Clinical Psychology & Psychotherapy, 16*(1), 55-76.

Dudley, R., Kuyken, W., & Padesky, C. A. (2011). Disorder specific and trans-diagnostic case conceptualisation. *Clinical Psychology Review, 31*(2), 213-224.

Elliott, R. (2002). Hermeneutic single-case efficacy design. *Psychotherapy Research, 12*(1), 1-21.

Ellis, A. (2004). Expanding the ABCs of Rational Emotive Behavior Therapy. In A. Freeman, M. J. Mahoney, P. Devito, & D. Martin (Eds.), *Cognition and psychotherapy* (2nd ed., pp. 185-195). New York: Springer.

Epley, N., Morewedge, C. K., & Keysar, B. (2004). Perspective taking in children and adults: Equivalent egocentrism but differential correction. *Journal of Experimental Social Psychology, 40*, 760-768.

Fennell, M. J. V. (1989). Depression. In K. Hawton, P. M. Salkovskis, J. Kirk, & D. M. Clark (Eds.), *Cognitive Behaviour Therapy for psychiatric problems* (pp. 169-234). Oxford: Oxford University Press.

Grant, A., Townend, M., Mills, J., & Cockx, A. (2008). *Assessment and case formulation in cognitive behavioural therapy*. London: Sage.

Hawton, K., Salkovskis, P. M., Kirk, J., & Clark, D. M. (1989). *Cognitive Behaviour Therapy for psychiatric problems*. Oxford: Oxford University Press.

Hayes, S. C., Villatte, M., Levin, M., & Hildebrandt, M. (2011). Open, aware, and active: Contextual approaches as an emerging trend in the behavioral and cognitive therapies. *Annual Review of Clinical Psychology, 7*, 141-168.

Hofmann, S. G., & Asmundson, G. J. (2008). Acceptance and mindfulness-based therapy: New wave or old hat? *Clinical Psychology Review, 28*(1), 1-16.

Hofmann, S. G., Asnaani, A., Vonk, I. J., Sawyer, A. T., & Fang, A. (2012). The efficacy of cognitive behavioral therapy: a review of meta-analyses. *Cognitive Therapy and Research, 36*(5), 427-440.

Jacobson, N. S., Dobson, K. S., Truax, P. A., Addis, M. E., Koerner, K., Gollan, J. K., . . . Prince, S. E. (1996). A component analysis of cognitive-behavioral treatment for depression. *Journal of Consulting and Clinical Psychology, 64*(2), 295-304.

Jacobson, N. S., & Truax, P. (1991). Clinical significance: A statistical approach to defining meaningful change in psychotherapy research. *Journal of Consulting and Clinical Psychology, 59*(1), 12-19.

Kazdin, A. E. (2009). Understanding how and why psychotherapy leads to change. *Psychotherapy Research, 19*(4-5), 418-428.

Knapp, P., & Beck, A. T. (2008). Fundamentos, modelos conceituais, aplicações e pesquisa da terapia cognitiva Cognitive therapy: foundations, conceptual models, applications and research. *Revista Brasileira de Psiquiatria, 30*(Supl II), S54-64.

Kuyken, W., Fothergill, C. D., Musa, M., & Chadwick, P. (2005). The reliability and quality of cognitive case formulation. *Behaviour Research and Therapy, 43*(9), 1187-1201.

Kuyken, W., Padesky, C. A., & Dudley, R. (2008). The science and practice of case conceptualization. *Behavioural and Cognitive Psychotherapy, 36*(06), 757-768.

Lemmens, L. H., Roefs, A., Arntz, A., van Teeseling, H. C., Peeters, F., & Huibers, M. J. (2014). The value of an implicit self-associative measure specific to core beliefs of depression. *Journal of Behavior Therapy and Experimental Psychiatry, 45*(1), 196-202.

Longmore, R. J., & Worrell, M. (2007). Do we need to challenge thoughts in cognitive behavior therapy? *Clinical Psychology Review, 27*(2), 173-187.

Morrison, A. P., & Barratt, S. (2010). What are the components of CBT for psychosis? A Delphi study. *Schizophrenia Bulletin, 36*(1), 136-142.

Mumma, G. H. (2004). Validation of idiosyncratic cognitive schema in cognitive case formulations: an intraindividual idiographic approach. *Psychological Assessment, 16*(3), 211-230.
Persons, J. B. (2008). *The case formulation approach to cognitive-behavior therapy*. New York: Guilford Press.
Rachman, S. (1981). The primacy of affect: Some theoretical implications. *Behaviour Research and Therapy, 19*(4), 279-290.
Rieckert, J., & Möller, A. T. (2000). Rational-Emotive Behavior Therapy in the treatment of adult victims of childhood sexual abuse. *Journal of Rational-Emotive & Cognitive-Behavior Therapy, 18*(2), 87-101.
Robertson, D. (2010). *The philosophy of cognitive-behavioural therapy (CBT): Stoic philosophy as rational and cognitive psychotherapy*. London: Karnac Books.
Ryan, R. M., Lynch, M. F., Vansteenkiste, M., & Deci, E. L. (2011). Motivation and autonomy in counseling, psychotherapy, and behavior change: A look at theory and practice. *The Counseling Psychologist, 39*(2), 193-260.
Storbeck, J., & Clore, G. L. (2007). On the interdependence of cognition and emotion. *Cognition and Emotion, 21*(6), 1212-1237.
Trickett, P. K., & McBride-Chang, C. (1995). The developmental impact of different forms of child abuse and neglect. *Developmental Review, 15*(3), 311-337.
Trower, P., Jones, J., Dryden, W., & Casey, A. (2011). *Cognitive behavioural counselling in action* (2nd ed.). London: Sage.

Aidan J P Hart

5 Acceptance and Commitment Therapy

This chapter will outline the detail and process of conducting a case formulation in Acceptance and Commitment Therapy (ACT – pronounced as a single word). The chapter will begin with a short description of the ACT model. Following this, the case of Molly will be discussed, and a preliminary formulation and treatment plan presented.

ACT is part of the wider family of cognitive and behavioural therapies, and is often considered to be part of the third wave of behavioural therapies. ACT builds upon classical and operant conditioning through a contemporary behavioural analysis of language and cognition (Relational Frame Theory; Hayes, Barnes-Holmes, & Roche, 2001). An account of the historical development of ACT can be found in Hayes, Strosahl and Wilson (1999) and a detailed introduction to Relational Frame Theory (RFT) can be found in Blackledge (2003) and Torneke (2010).

5.1 Defining Features

ACT rests on a small number of core principles: (1) psychological pain is normal and experienced by everyone; (2) pain and suffering are not the same thing; (3) we cannot deliberately get rid of our pain, and attempts to do so may actually amplify our suffering; (4) accepting pain is the first step towards reducing suffering; (5) psychological pain does not need to disappear in order to lead a life that one values; (6) distress is a function of context: There is nothing faulty, broken, or maladaptive 'inside' the client.

ACT makes a distinction between 'pain' and 'suffering': 'pain' is the normal emotional distress that one experiences in the course of life; 'suffering', on the other hand, is the additional distress experienced as a result of attempts to avoid or control pain. Consider a person who experiences a fear of rejection. Consequently they avoid relationships in order to reduce their fear (pain). However, as a result of avoiding relationships, the person may experience loneliness, isolation, and a life other than the one that they want to live. In this case, the pain of the fear of rejection is being managed by avoidance of relationships, which leads to the suffering of loneliness and isolation. From an ACT perspective our target is reducing suffering and building a better life through the acceptance of pain.

Because ACT is not focused on reduction of pain *per se*, we are not primarily interested in symptom reduction either (although this may be a secondary gain). Instead, we are interested in 'growing the person' rather than 'shrinking the problem'. While it is tempting to wish to reduce the person's problems and/or symptoms directly, ACT aims to 'expand' individuals so that they are enabled to live a life characterised by whatever matters to them, whilst highlighting that one's pain need not reduce or disappear in order for a meaningful life to be lived.

5.1.1 Experiential Avoidance and Psychological Flexibility

Experiential avoidance is defined within the ACT model as an active unwillingness to experience certain private events, such as thoughts, emotions, and physical sensations (Hayes, Wilson, Gifford, Follette, & Strosahl, 1996). ACT proposes that such avoidance not only amplifies those events but takes a person away from the life they wish to live. The ACT model makes a pragmatic distinction between helpful and unhelpful avoidance: If avoidance leads to an increase in pain, brings other problems into one's life, or takes one away from the life that they want, then we would consider such avoidance to be unhelpful.

ACT seeks to replace experiential avoidance with psychological flexibility. Psychological flexibility is the ability to connect with the present moment – fully, as a conscious human being – and to engage in behaviour that is consistent with personally-identified values (Hayes et al., 1999). In a context where avoidance of psychological pain has not worked, is not working, and will not work, ACT advocates acceptance as an alternative strategy that can help individuals to take action in accordance with their values. Therefore, ACT could be summarised by the three statements: (1) accept those experiences that you cannot avoid, (2) choose where you want to go in life, and (3) take action to that end.

This is of course not as simple as it sounds. In ACT, as in all therapeutic interventions, we ask the client to go on a difficult journey with us, and this should not be underestimated or trivialised.

5.2 Core Processes

ACT proposes that there are six core processes that underpin psychological wellbeing and flexibility: acceptance; cognitive defusion; contact with the present moment; self-as-context; values; and committed action. These processes are conceptualised as being interconnected: they are not considered to be standalone processes to be worked through sequentially. Due to their interconnected nature, it is not uncommon for a typical ACT session to focus on several of these processes.

5.2.1 Acceptance

Acceptance from an ACT perspective is not resignation; it is does not mean tolerating the intolerable or giving in – these are fatalistic and passive responses. Acceptance also does not preclude obvious workable solutions to problems, such as making beneficial changes to one's environment. Instead, acceptance refers to an active and engaging stance that is true to its etymological root meaning: "take what is offered" (Hayes & Strosahl, 2004). In this context, acceptance is a stance of actively and non-judgementally embracing whatever thoughts, emotions, and physical feelings one experiences, when avoidance is not working. This is of course much harder than might be suggested by these few brief sentences. Often clients will come to therapy having tried for years to avoid painful thoughts and feelings. Some clients would rather be in abusive relationships than experience loneliness; some would rather be intoxicated or cut and burn themselves than think or feel. The difficulty of acceptance should not be underestimated.

Acceptance is fostered by helping clients to experientially contact the costs of avoidance. It is hoped that clients see that, with respect to private events (thoughts, feelings, and sensations), avoidance or control is often the problem and not the solution. Clients are encouraged to confront the unworkability or costliness of avoidance and control in an empathic and non-self-blaming manner. The futility of avoidance, suppression, and control is highlighted so as to create space for new possibilities. Simple brief exercises and metaphors such as 'Tug of War with a Monster' (Hayes et al., 1999; p.101) can be used to make these points effectively. This metaphor presents the client with the conundrum that they are engaged in a 'tug of war' with their psychological pain (the 'monster'). No matter how hard they struggle, the monster pulls harder, prompting ever greater effort from the client. What we want the client to realise is that the first step here must be to drop the rope. This is to help create a space in which alternatives to struggling can be experienced. This metaphor is similar to the concept of 'trying to dig yourself out of a hole': It does not matter how you got there, digging further certainly does not help you to escape; the first step is to lay down the shovel. It is important to recognise that avoidance can often be effective in the short-term, and clients may consequently have a strong reinforcement history for avoidance behaviour. Even for clients who recognise that their avoidance is not very effective in the longer-term, there may be a strong element of negative reinforcement at work in that their avoidance may be keeping larger threats and 'scarier monsters' at bay.

5.2.2 Cognitive Defusion

Humans have a tendency to respond to thoughts as if they are the 'thing thought about' as opposed to a verbal or visual representation of it. When remembering and thinking about a past negative experience, clients will respond (most likely at a lower level of intensity) in a manner similar to when they directly experienced the event itself (e.g., fear, anxiety, or shame), even though the tangible properties of the experience are no longer present; this phenomenon is known within ACT as *cognitive fusion* (for a more comprehensive discussion of this process from an RFT perspective, see Blackledge,

2003; Torneke, 2010). Thoughts are not problematic in and of themselves (Hayes & Strosahl, 2004), but may become a problem or a barrier to effective change if they are afforded weight or particular significance by the individual experiencing them. In ACT, we help the person to develop a different *relationship* with their thoughts by employing cognitive defusion exercises.

The purpose of cognitive defusion is to help clients view and experience their thoughts as not being 'literal truths' but rather psychological experiences that can be acted upon – or not. Whether the thought is 'true' is not considered to be the key issue; instead, the focus is on how one responds to the thought. In this regard, ACT is different from traditional forms of cognitive behavioural therapy (CBT) in that cognitive restructuring is not used and the thought is not engaged with or challenged at the level of content. For example, a client might report to the therapist that they think that no one likes them. The therapist would not ask for evidence for or against the thought, but might instead ask the client "if you buy into that thought, if you respond as if it is true, where does that take you?" Here an ACT therapist is attempting to get the client to reflect upon the 'life-narrowing' implications of acting on the thought as if it were true. Cognitive defusion interventions may utilise 'physicalizing' and externalising exercises to promote a shift in the context and function of thoughts. For example, a client may be asked to take a negative self-referential thought or label and to imagine putting the thought out in front of them on the floor and to begin to describe its 'physical' properties. The function of such exercises is to loosen the client's attachment to their thoughts, re-contextualising the experience of thinking, and to begin to create space between the person and their thoughts. A further way of changing the contextual experience of thoughts is to use a technique borrowed from Gestalt psychology. A word with eliciting properties is repeated over and over, faster and faster until the person notices a change in the sensations elicited. Other techniques might be to say the negative thoughts in a silly voice (a favourite of the late great Albert Ellis). It should be noted that such changes in function are likely to be temporary and the purpose here is not to elicit a permanent change in the response to thoughts, or to belittle or ridicule the client's thinking, but to *practice* responding differently to thoughts whilst refraining from attempts to change their content.

5.2.3 Contact With the Present Moment

The purpose of acceptance and cognitive defusion is to enable a client to 'show up' to the present moment in the service of connecting to personal values and living in accordance with them. Contact with the present moment is strongly connected to the process and stance of acceptance in that it functions to promote effective and undefended contact with whatever is happening in the 'here and now'. This is important, because in order for a client to decide how best to respond to a given situation, the client must be present and in contact with it.

Clients are helped to label and describe experiences without excessive and unhelpful evaluation and judgement. Teaching clients to be present helps foster acceptance and to stay in the 'here and now' where workable solutions are to be found. This does not mean that clients are discouraged from remembering past events or from thinking forward to the future; it is when the 'hold' of such thinking takes the client away from living life in the present that it becomes problematic.

One of the main ways in which contact with the present moment is fostered is with a variety of mindfulness and orientation (or 'noticing') exercises. In such exercises, clients are simply orientated to whatever physical feelings, sensations, thoughts or emotions are showing up for them at a given time, without getting caught up in them.

5.2.4 Self as Context (Over Content)

Self as context is strongly connected to the process of cognitive defusion in that both processes contend with the literality of language and other private content. Self as context processes are designed to help clients distinguish and separate out from their conceptualised selves (i.e., self as *content*). Key messages in any self as context work are (1) that you are not your thoughts, your emotions, or your memories; and (2) that there is a *you*, a bigger you (the context), wherein such things happen (i.e., where private content occurs). We want clients to experience – if only for a moment – that there is a place from which such things can be experienced, a place where such things cannot hurt them. An ACT therapist will help a client experience self as context in a number of ways. For example, through the use of mindfulness exercises where clients are helped to experience their thoughts and feelings as an observer. The therapist might also use simple metaphors to help the client make a distinction between themselves and their content. Such metaphors may include: "you are the house not the furniture, the chessboard not the pieces, the sky not the clouds".

5.2.5 Values

Clients in therapy are often stuck in patterns of behaviour that are about controlling and eliminating unwanted private events rather than leading a life full of personal meaning. ACT seeks to help clients regain this life-direction; however, it is important to remember that many clients will not have given consideration to what they value or want out of life. Some clients arrive in therapy from a place where they have not been permitted to even think about such things, and some will therefore inevitably struggle to think about them now. Despite this, it can often be useful to enquire about values early in assessment and treatment. ACT, like many other psychological therapies, involves clients contacting experiences and physical places that they have been avoiding. Change is therefore difficult and there has to be some perceived and anticipated benefit or reinforcement for making change. Whilst the client may be understandably focussed on reduction of symptoms, values work speaks to what this reduction is for (if you were to feel less anxious, what would you be doing then?). Values assessment also sends a message to the client that therapy will contain a space for the things that they love and care about, and a focus on how to begin having more of such things.

Values clarification in ACT takes place through questioning and experiential exercises. Clients can be asked questions like "if you could have your life stand for anything, what would you choose it to stand for?" Clients may also be asked to imagine a speech given about them at a ceremony honouring their life achievements; what would they like to hear?

It is important to make a distinction with clients between values and goals. The purpose of values is not necessarily the achievement of specific goals. Values can be thought of as signposts: A common metaphor used in ACT work is that living in line with one's values is like traveling west. One never reaches 'west' as a destination, but can continue travelling west indefinitely. Many things can be experienced and achieved whilst travelling in ones chosen direction; it is the journey and not the destination that is important. From a behavioural perspective, values speak to the function of goals and give an idea to the therapist of sources of reinforcement for future behavioural activation. One of the advantages of understanding such functions is that it can help the therapist guide committed action (see below) towards a variety of goals. It can also help a client find new goals should one become unavailable to them. An extreme example could be the loss of a job or a cherished role through injury. While a person may not be able to continue in their previous role, if we know the value – i.e., the function of their role, and what it was that made the role important – we can help the client find other ways to stay connected to that value.

5.2.6 Committed Action

ACT is at heart a behavioural treatment and as such the previous five processes above serve to elicit actual change in the client's behaviour to serve valued ends. All other processes in ACT therapy lead to this point, and the client, knowing that avoidance is not working, and knowing what they want from life, has to decide to commit to change and to actively implement it. Living and acting in line with one's values is the context in which acceptance is worthwhile.

Like most effective behavioural exercises, committed action starts with smaller goals, similar to graded exposure or graded behavioural activation. Once a client has started on their path of values-guided behavioural change, it is expected that natural reinforcement will occur to maintain the change. It is important at this stage to prepare clients for problems that may surface and barriers that may arise. Often when a client commits to valued living they may predict failure and experience anxiety (loss of contact with the present), or they may believe they will fail because they are inadequate (cognitive fusion and self as context). Clients can be prepared for this, by letting them know that their mind will not want change and may fight back, or that their anxiety or depression will fight for its survival (this represents a defusion metaphor in itself). Clients are asked to consider questions such as "what pain would you be willing to have in order to do what you love and care about?"

5.3 Evidence Base

ACT is an emerging and developing therapeutic approach and over the last 15 years has strengthened its evidence-base considerably. To date, ACT has been used successfully in the treatment of depression, anxiety, OCD, chronic pain, diabetes management, and psychosis, and its efficacy is discussed in a number of published positive reviews from Hayes, Luoma, Bond, Masuda, and Lillis (2006), Gaudiano (2009), Levin and Hayes (2009), and Ruiz (2010, 2012). More critical reviews have been published by Öst (2008, 2014) and by Powers, Zum Vörde Sive Vörding, and Emmelkamp (2009).

5.4 Formulation in Action

An ACT case conceptualisation will typically involve six activities on the part of the therapist (Hayes & Strosahl, 2004): (1) assess the scope and nature of the presenting problem; (2) identify the experiences that the client is attempting to avoid; (3) identify behaviours/methods that the client is using to facilitate their avoidance; (4) assess the factors that may be reducing motivation for change; (5) assess and identify any environmental barriers to change; and (6) consider factors likely to be contributing to inflexibility (e.g., fusion, self as content, domination of the past/future, values uncertainty, low levels of committed action).

5.4.1 Assess the Scope and Nature of the Presenting Problem

Molly appears to have learned to avoid situations that elicit anxiety or other negative experiences. Her history with other people is also likely to have contributed to Molly developing negative self-labels, and importantly, to accept these labels as 'true' (self-as-content and fusion). Her attempts to avoid situations that elicit anxiety or negative thoughts/self-labelling appears to be hindering her ability to live her life in a way that is meaningful to her (i.e., a lack of valued direction or valued action).

Molly states that she "wants to get better", "feel the opposite of how she does now", "feel more confident", and "make everyone proud". From an ACT perspective this is a mix of both appetitive and avoidance goals. I would be keen to know what "getting better" means for her: what would she be able to do if she were better? This is similar to the 'miracle question' often asked in Solution Focused Approaches (i.e., what would the client's life be like if perceived problems were no longer present; De Jong & Berg, 2012). It is likely at this stage that the issue of wanting to be "more confident" would arise. In a similar manner, I would want to know what she would do if she were more confident and would hypothesise that Molly's lack of confidence may manifest in predictions of future failure – indeed, she mentions twice that there is "no point" attempting to improve her situation. The anticipation of failure is likely to be emotionally distressing, and Molly may attempt to reduce her distress by eliminating the possibility of failure (e.g., by simply 'not doing'). As these issues emerged during therapy, I would offer ACT-informed observations of Molly's self-report. For example, if Molly describes an anticipation of future failure, I might respond thus:

Molly: There is no point trying, it won't work; it never does.
Therapist: It sounds like every time you want something better or try for something better, your mind comes in and tells you it will be bad, not to bother. Then what happens?
Molly: I begin to get worried, I feel anxious and scared and I think 'what's the point?' so I don't bother.
Therapist: So when you believe what your mind tells you and you do what it says where does that leave you?
Molly: Well, I feel less worried about the future.
Therapist: But here and now?
Molly: Here and now I just feel stupid and useless for not trying and I'm still stuck where I don't want to be.

While in actuality, the above exchange rarely (if ever) happens so neatly, it hopefully illustrates the point. What I would be attempting to do through this process is to help Molly gain awareness of the cycle she is stuck in and the manner in which her avoidance not only keeps her away from a future that she wants, but also makes her more miserable in the present. The use of language such as "your mind comes in and tells you" is deliberate and is designed to facilitate defusion at a later stage by beginning to encourage Molly to consider her mind as almost like a separate entity – and one that is not necessarily acting in her best interests.

I also get a sense that Molly might be playing a 'waiting game' with her emotions. She might be waiting for things to get better or for her to feel different before she can move on with her life. This is of course understandable, given her experience of the world to date. I would, however, begin to explore with Molly the possibility that the waiting game may not work. I would want Molly to begin to consider that, rather than waiting for these experiences to disappear before she starts living her life, she can begin to live and take these experiences along with her.

5.4.2 Identify what Experiences the Client is Attempting to Avoid

Many of the experiences that Molly seems to be avoiding could be classified under a larger umbrella of fear of rejection/abandonment by her parents and her peers. Connected to this, Molly is also troubled by thoughts and beliefs about her own unworthiness, incompetence, and unattractiveness – and the expectation that she will fail at everything she does. She is also suffering from the impact of being sexually abused when she was nine years old. We would hypothesise that, due to the effects of classical conditioning, sex and sexual intimacy may now function as a conditioned aversive. As such, it seems that she is now avoiding intimate sexual relationships. It is also likely she is 'fused' with the memories of the abuse to an extent where thinking about the abuse, or thinking about sex, may elicit distressing emotional and physiological responses.

5.4.3 What Behaviours/Methods is the Client Using to Facilitate Their Avoidance?

There are a number of ways in which Molly has avoided or attempted to avoid these negative experiences. Molly's avoidance seems to be facilitated by physically avoiding situations and contexts, and also by being overly compliant with her parents. It can be seen from the case description that Molly maintains a close proximity to her parents and does many things for them that they are capable of doing for themselves. I would hypothesise that, given her historical experiences within the family, Molly is attempting to avoid painful feelings relating to thoughts of being unlovable and taking second place to her sister.

Molly also avoids social contact with others and as a result lives a somewhat reclusive lifestyle. She has been let down by others in the past and fears their rejection and ridicule. As a result, she is likely to predict that other people will mistreat her or reject her in some way. Consequently, she avoids the anticipatory negative emotions by avoiding or minimising her social relationships; or by having them online where she may be able to maintain a larger degree of control over them. It is also likely that Molly's avoidance of romantic and sexual relationships is a function of her sexual abuse experiences. Her descriptions of her relationship with Danny indicate that her difficulty in being intimate with him could be a function of her abuse experiences. Her reluctance to have further relationships could also serve the function of reducing her contact with these feelings.

5.4.4 Assess the Factors That May be Reducing Motivation for Change

While Molly gives indications of what she wants, there may still be factors inhibiting her motivation for change; in particular, her predictions of future failure. Molly's descriptions of her past indicate a number of aversive experiences, which have arisen while pursuing apparent valued ends. University did not work out; similarly, her job as a teaching assistant did not progress, and her current role at the library is also not as she would wish. Similarly, her experiences of sexual and romantic relationships have been negative. One of the biggest barriers to change for Molly will be her expectation that change is not possible or that she is not capable of change – and the anxiety and fear that this elicits. From an ACT perspective, Molly is heavily fused with her low opinion of herself and her expectations that she can only fail.

5.4.5 Assess any Environmental Barriers to Change

Superficially, Molly appears to have access to a number of resources, such as her job and her own accommodation, which may help to facilitate change. However, one external barrier to change for Molly is likely to be found in her relationship with her parents. If Molly is to make progress then it is likely that her relationship with her parents will need to change also. Despite being physically able, Molly's parents have come to depend on her to run errands for them, and Molly reports that they make her feel guilty if she does not meet their demands. The reaction of Molly's parents is likely to be an environmental barrier; from her description, I would predict that should she change the nature of her relationship with them (i.e., by doing less for them) then it is likely that they will put additional pressure on her to keep the status quo. In such a context, I would be mindful of the likely negative judgements Molly might make about herself, the feelings of guilt that might arise, and would target these in treatment.

5.4.6 Consider the Factors Contributing to Psychological Inflexibility

Factors contributing to inflexibility are presented in Table 5.1.

Table 5.1: Sources of inflexibility for Molly

Source of inflexibility	Presenting difficulties
Areas avoided	Molly avoids socialising with others. She avoids contact at work (as she did her house mates when a student) and has few friends. She prefers to socialise online. Molly also avoids confronting her parents about their treatment of her and avoids telling them about her sexual abuse. Further to this, Molly avoids intimate sexual relationships and is no longer pursuing her dream of being a teacher.
Cognitive entanglement (fusion and self-as-content)	Molly believes that she is unlovable, unworthy, unattractive, and unable to succeed at what she wants. She also defines herself by her mental health problems: she is fused with the stigma of having been in the 'nuthouse' and believes that her parents must see her as a 'freak show'. Molly also feels 'dirty' and self-judgemental whenever she has sexual thoughts or sexual contact with another person.
Domination of the past/ future	There is some evidence from the information provided that Molly finds it difficult to remain in the 'present moment'. For Molly the present moment and her current context seem to be dominated by aversive stimuli: She is relatively socially isolated, has negative relationships with her family, and is constantly reminded of past abuses (sexual abuse), rejections (boyfriends), and academic and occupational failures (university).
Values uncertainty	There is some evidence that Molly identifies some personal values, but these appear fairly limited to a specific area (e.g. work/teaching). Although wanting to be a teacher is a goal rather than a value, it is likely to be directed by some core values, and this would be explored further. Molly also presents with behaviours that *ap*pear to be values-driven but which may not be: She undertakes a lot for her parents who are quite capable, and it is possible that this is driven by a need to feel useful and loved by them, or more accurately, a need to avoid feeling unloved. Whilst efforts to evade 'feeling unloved' are of course understandable, the risk for Molly is that she gives her life over to avoiding such feelings – to the detriment of what she wants for herself. It would seem that her relationship with her sister and her friend Eve is a potential area for development.
Low levels of committed Action	Molly appears to engage in little values-guided activity at present and this would be a key area for development.

5.4.7 Intervention Objectives

The following outlines areas for potential intervention; however, it is not necessarily reflective of the order in which work would be undertaken, nor should it be understood that the interventions would be implemented in a separate, serial manner. It is also worth remembering that the boundaries between assessment and intervention may be more blurred in ACT, and that aspects of normalisation and values work are likely to come up at various times during the assessment. Likewise, having the client discuss difficulties and unworkable change strategies inherently involves elements of exposure, defusion, and movement towards acceptance, and these aspects would be visited, and revisited, throughout my work with Molly.

5.4.7.1 Normalisation

One of the first treatment goals or strategies I would introduce for Molly would be a normalisation of her experience. Molly seems stuck in a cycle of avoidance that is consuming her life to the extent that I do not have a full sense of where she wants to go: what she wants her life to 'stand for', in ACT parlance. Even though she will undoubtedly be experiencing many negative self-appraisals and be engaged in counter-productive avoidance strategies, I would want Molly to know that this is a normal response to her situation. I would begin to highlight areas of 'fusion' and begin to reflect these back using defusion techniques (e.g., 'what is your mind telling you?'). In addition to normalising her experience, by beginning to talk about her mind in this way, we are attempting to create some distance between Molly and her 'private content'. Whilst not advocating a dualist position, we are pragmatically helping Molly to separate out and step back from her psychological content, and I would deliberately speak in these terms throughout the assessment and intervention. The second aspect of the normalisation stage would be to consider the avoidance strategies that Molly is using. Again, I would have a discussion around the pull of avoidance, and how it is ultimately ineffective when it comes to our private experiences. I would be extremely careful that Molly does not feel blamed for being stuck, and this conversation would be had in the context of an understanding that avoidance is something that we all practice. The function of these discussions would be to highlight to Molly that she is not intrinsically or internally broken, but that she is currently stuck as a result of how she has been taught to 'play the game' (e.g. that aversive experiences need to be avoided or overcome before meaningful action can be undertaken). I would conclude by highlighting that, while the road ahead will be a difficult one, I will do everything I can to help her to get her life moving again.

5.4.7.2 Values

Whilst the majority of the work on values and associated behavioural activation goals would come later in therapy, I would typically also start to discuss values early on. When asked about 'values' early in therapy, many clients are unable to answer. This might be because they simply don't know: They have been so busy surviving that they have not had the opportunity to think about it. In other cases, clients may have had to subjugate their own needs to those of others; or may have an active history of being punished for attempting to live their own values. Most (if not all) of these experiences are likely to apply to Molly in some way, affording her little opportunity to clarify personal values. Consequently, Molly may be somewhat perplexed and resistant when asked about her own values. Despite this, my experience suggests that it is an important area to explore at an early stage for the following reasons: (1) I want Molly to know that she has the possibility of a brighter future guided by the things that she cares about; (2) I want Molly to know that the difficult journey I am going to ask her to take is going somewhere important to her; and (3) I want Molly to know that, whilst therapy will involve discussion about and contact with things that are painful, there will still be space for the things that she loves, cherishes, and values.

5.4.7.3 Acceptance

When working with Molly, I would help her to contact and to appreciate the costs of her struggle, and the unworkability of avoidance. This should be done in the context of the normalisation described above. It is important that Molly is not blamed for being stuck; the message that she is doing as life has taught her comes to the fore, and there is no blame to be apportioned. This does not, however, preclude Molly from experiencing self-judgmental thoughts about her situation. In fact, the case material as presented would lead me to hypothesise that these experiences would occur for Molly. This is why the language of defusion should run though the assessment and the intervention, allowing the therapist to identify such negative judgements and to externalise them as the 'mind' being unhelpful. An important aspect of acceptance-focussed work is to examine the larger cost of avoidance, in that it can take us away from our values and our goals. This is why I often find it useful to have the conversation on values early on; it creates a context in which there is a benefit to at least considering acceptance as a workable alternative to avoidance.

5.4.7.4 Contact With the Present Moment

There are indications that Molly's ability to contact the present moment is undermined by the dominance of the past. She conveys the ongoing impact of previous difficulties – her relationship with her family, being seen as second best to her sister, the experience of being sexually abused, failed relationships, and problems with work and education. I get a sense that these past events have come to occupy Molly and interfere with her ability to take effective action in the here and now. Using mindfulness techniques, I would want Molly to be able to differentiate between 'then' and 'now', in an attempt to lessen her fusion with the past, so as to foster values-consistent action in the present.

5.4.7.5 Defusion and Self-as-Context

This part of therapy is where ACT takes a more distinctive approach to other interventions within the broader cognitive and behavioural family. As mentioned in the summary above, the emphasis in ACT is on acceptance of private events rather than change or elimination of them. In this element of the treatment I would work with Molly to loosen the control that such experiences have on her. This would hopefully lead to Molly being able to see her thoughts 'as thoughts as opposed to facts'. The content of the thought is not challenged or evidence tested, but Molly is instead asked to consider how useful the thought is for her life plan (this again points to the utility of developing knowledge of her values at an early point in therapy).

A large part of this work would focus on her experiences of sexual abuse and the negative judgements that she makes about herself in relation to these experiences. In this element of treatment, I would of course not be seeking to stop her thinking about the abuse, or even to reduce the occurrence of abuse-related memories, but more to reduce the impact of remembering when it does inevitably occur. We can see from her descriptions of connecting sex to labels such as "dirty" that there is a dominant impact of her abuse experiences in the present. At a purely technical level, the impact of these experiences would be tackled in the same manner as other negative private content. The scope and nature of the abuse would form part of the initial assessment, in as much as she is willing to discuss it, and it may be that such work is left to later in the treatment.

5.4.7.6 Goal Orientation and Committed Action

During this phase of therapy I would begin by returning to the concept of values in more detail. Molly has reported good relationships with her sister and her friend Eva and there is a strong sense that 'being a teacher' has been of value to her in the past. This in particular is evident from her working as a classroom assistant. However, as part of our assessment and treatment, we need to make a distinction between Molly's own values and goals versus those that may come from her family's expectations of her. If Molly pursuing a career in teaching was an example of the latter, then this may indicate a degree of aversive control and suggest that her aspirations in this domain may be more about avoiding the disapproval of her family.

It is unclear whether Molly wishes to have another romantic or sexual relationship; however, the manner in which she discusses this area of her life indicates issues that require further exploration. She provides reasons as to why it would be 'pointless' to pursue future relationships, rather than stating this is something she does not want or value. This seems to me to be the expression of a value or goal being blocked, as opposed to something that is not valued. In this phase of therapy, I would help Molly to identify goals in line with her values, and collaboratively build a graded hierarchy of value-based activities for her to engage in during therapy.

5.4.7.7 Treatment Summary

1. Normalise and contextualise her experience; highlight that she is not 'damaged' or 'broken', but rather 'stuck';
2. Identify and clarify her values and associated goals, and begin to identify the internal and external barriers to pursuing them;
3. Use cognitive defusion and self-as context strategies to loosen the control and dominance of private experiences;
4. Use mindfulness to facilitate exposure to private experiences and encourage present moment awareness;
5. Build patterns of committed action relevant to her values, employing skills training (e.g., assertiveness with her parents) where needed.

5.4.8 Measuring Effectiveness

Given that ACT as an approach is not focused on symptom reduction, how do we therefore measure the effectiveness of our interventions? Within an ACT model, we measure success by how much a client is reengaged with and living the life that she/he wants, loves, values, and cares about. In Molly's case, I would hope that she would be able to assert her needs with her parents, doing less for them and more for herself. I would hope to see spending more time in the company of others, and perhaps with her friend Eva in particular. I would also hope to see Molly happier in her current job, or pursuing a career more relevant to her personal values. A final area in which I would hope to see Molly make progress would be in respect to the impact of the sexual abuse on her life, particularly its apparent effect on her ability to form new intimate relationships. If developing a new relationship was identified as being consistent with Molly's values, then we would look for evidence of this when assessing therapeutic gains.

Kerry Beckley

5.5 ACT Formulation: Critical Commentary

ACT aims to pragmatically facilitate a person to cope in the here and now, by accepting life as it is and building towards a more value-orientated future. The evidence-base thus far appears to demonstrate moderate effect sizes for a range of less complex mental health problems. However, Öst (2008) conducted a meta-analysis of RCTs of third wave behavioural therapies and concluded that ACT could not be considered an empirically supported treatment. ACT has been criticised for not using diagnostic categories in half of the studies of clinical effectiveness, and some studies also appear to have less methodological stringency in comparison to more general CBT RCTs in terms of: reliability and validity of outcome measures, number of therapists and level of therapist training, statistical analysis, presentation of results, equality of therapy hours, diagnostic adherence, and checks on treatment adherence.

The central tenet of 'growing the person' as opposed to 'shrinking the problem' is an attractive clinical prospect but it is not one which, by itself, is proven to be effective with more complex and sustained mental health presentations such as personality disorder. Arguably, this idea is not solely the domain of third wave behavioural therapies, and parallels can be drawn with the behavioural pattern-breaking aspects of Schema Therapy (ST; Young, Klosko & Weishaar, 2003) in the growth of the Healthy Adult Mode. Both approaches make use of meta-cognitive interventions to weaken the relationship between deeply rooted ideas of self and others. The approaches appear to differ most in terms of the assumed aetiology of the client's difficulties, the importance of content and language in terms of creating opportunities for change, and the explicit use of the therapeutic relationship within therapy.

There is, however, a significant degree of similarity in the formulations of Molly presented from apparently opposing theoretical positions. ACT uses the term 'avoidance' as an overarching concept which would encompass all three coping strategies seen in the ST model. Both approaches would view past experiences in terms of their reinforcing attributes; ST would place less assumption on Molly 'knowing' what she really wants, but would understand her schema-reinforcing actions as ways of sustaining a sense of self and other that is familiar. The use of defusion within the therapy exchange parallels the idea of separating the 'Punitive/Demanding' Parent Modes from the person; in contrast to ST, ACT uses this separation to enable clients to question and be more sceptical of their thoughts. However, it is not clear what happens next if this is not effective. ST would consider that intervention by the therapist is crucial: the therapist would align with Molly to enable her to have an experience of someone standing up to her internalised critical self, whilst supporting her in weakening the influence it has on her.

Both formulations highlight Molly's fear of abandonment/rejection, linked to her own sense of unworthiness and failure. The ACT formulation goes further in its consideration of the impact of sexual abuse. Although the hypothesised impact has merit, it may be premature in its assumption that Molly finds sex distressing, given the other factors which contribute to her avoidance of close relationships. Molly's barriers to change are formulated in similar ways: that her repeated experiences of failure have resulted in her predicting that her future holds more of the same. However, the ACT formulation extends further by explicitly predicting that Molly's parents may present an environmental barrier to change (negative external feedback as she begins to do less for them). ST would place more emphasis on the development and maintenance of a stable sense of self and other, that is resilient to the demands placed on us by others.

Both treatments similarly take the form of a set of *principles*, rather than a set of interventions, which are undertaken in a linear fashion. Like ST, ACT attempts to normalise avoidance (given Molly's history) and uses strategies to create distance between Molly and her ‘private content’. The therapeutic language in both models, although different in content, is crucial in achieving this. The idea of being ‘stuck’ because of how she has been taught to ‘play the game’ parallels the ideas in ST of strategies which previously had protective value to survive trauma, but now continue as though the client was still in that set of circumstances.

The ACT formulation highlights the role of the therapist as facilitator, but there is far less emphasis on the therapeutic relationship. For individuals who have significant difficulties in the relational domain, this appears to be a weakness of the outlined intervention. Molly’s template of ‘other’ as rejecting/uninterested is likely to permeate the therapeutic relationship and impede the aims of the intervention unless explicitly worked with.

ACT places emphasis on the space to consider values in therapy, which may differ somewhat from ST’s emphasis on unmet needs, but in essence they are aiming to achieve the same outcome. Those who work in an integrative way with both approaches have highlighted how this more explicit focus on ACT principles and interventions can augment aspects of ST: suggesting that, with more complex presentations, change-focused work may first be necessary, before acknowledging that some things cannot be changed and should therefore be accepted (Roediger, 2012). A strength of the ACT model is the importance of keeping Molly’s values central to the therapeutic narrative and how this can be utilised in developing value-based tasks for homework. It makes intuitive sense that a client would be more likely to engage in activities which aim to enhance enjoyment and purpose, than to directly work on a task which aims to reduce something they actively avoid. This is also true of the measurements of success, which ultimately reflect Molly’s values rather than symptom reduction – which may or may not lead to improvements in her quality of life.

Aidan J P Hart

5.6 Author Response

This seems to a reasonably fair summary and critique of the model and formulation as presented in the chapter. There are two areas of the critique I would like to address: the issue of sexual abuse and the therapeutic relationship.

I would accept that the focus in the formulation on sexual abuse may indeed be premature, and I acknowledge that more information is certainly required. A formulation is of course a working hypothesis that is always subject to revision. As such, it might be that the formulation is revised with respect to sexual abuse, if further exploration suggests that this experience does not appear central to Molly’s current difficulties.

In my experience of delivering ACT training, a question often asked is how an individual could be expected to simply ‘accept’ abuse. By including the sexual abuse in the formulation, I was attempting to offer an example of how one might conceptualise this experience within the ACT assessment, formulation, and treatment framework. This is not to say that it would always be included in this manner, or indeed at all.

The main aspect of the critique I would like to address is the point about the therapeutic relationship. ACT by no means minimises the importance of the therapeutic relationship in facilitating client change. From a pragmatic point of view, if the client does not trust or value the therapist, or if the therapist is experienced negatively, then therapy will inevitably be impeded. The therapeutic relationship is important, first and foremost, because if the client in not in the room with the therapist, and does not return for further sessions, then the therapist cannot help them. It is important that a humanising, supportive, and safe environment is created that helps maximise the client's commitment to change whilst minimising any coercion on the part of the therapist (Hayes & Strosahl, 2004). This is not a new concept from a behavioural point of view, and can be found in the notion of the therapist as a 'non-punishing audience' (Skinner, 1953; see Chapter 3).

The importance of the therapeutic relationship is not just limited to keeping the client in the room, however, but is central to every aspect of the ACT process. The relationship in ACT is a fully collaborative one. A key message is that the therapist is not immune to the processes of experiential avoidance, fusion, etc. To that end, the therapist will often talk about ACT processes with the client in the context of "we" rather than exclusively "you". In an ACT intervention, the therapist will communicate hope and optimism for change, and a passionate interest in helping the client to pursue their values. The therapist will also use the context of the therapeutic relationship to model ACT-relevant processes – and experiential exposure in particular.

A final reason why the therapeutic relationship is important is connected to the fact that a large part of ACT is dedicated to breaking down patterns of avoidance and exposure to feared interoceptive and exteroceptive stimuli; this is often difficult for the client to engage in, and a meaningful and trusting therapeutic relationship is essential. In my experience, in the context of a strong empathic therapeutic relationship, clients will go to the difficult places that are necessary as part of the therapeutic journey, and will forgive you most mistakes you may make along the way. Without the foundational bedrock of a good therapeutic relationship, then the rest of the model becomes largely unworkable.

References

Blackledge, J. T. (2003). An introduction to relational frame theory: Basics and applications. *The Behavior Analyst Today, 3*(4), 421-433.

De Jong, P., & Berg, I. K. (2012). *Interviewing for solutions*. Belmont, CA: Cengage Learning.

Gaudiano, B. A. (2009). Öst's (2008) methodological comparison of clinical trials of acceptance and commitment therapy versus cognitive behavior therapy: Matching Apples with Oranges? *Behaviour Research and Therapy, 47*(12), 1066-1070.

Hayes, S. C., Barnes-Holmes, D., & Roche, B. (2001). *Relational Frame Theory: A Post-Skinnerian account of human language and cognition*. New York: Plenum Press.

Hayes, S. C., Luoma, J. B., Bond, F. W., Masuda, A., & Lillis, J. (2006). Acceptance and commitment therapy: Model, processes and outcomes. *Behaviour Research and Therapy, 44*(1), 1-25.

Hayes, S. C., & Strosahl, K. (2004). *A practical guide to Acceptance and Commitment Therapy*. New York: Springer.

Hayes, S. C., Strosahl, K., & Wilson, K. G. (1999). *Acceptance and Commitment Therapy: An experiential approach to behavior change*. New York: Guilford Press.

Hayes, S. C., Wilson, K. G., Gifford, E. V., Follette, V. M., & Strosahl, K. (1996). Experiential avoidance and behavioral disorders: A functional dimensional approach to diagnosis and treatment. *Journal of Consulting and Clinical Psychology, 64*(6), 1152-1168.

Levin, M., & Hayes, S. C. (2009). Is Acceptance and commitment therapy superior to established treatment comparisons? *Psychotherapy and Psychosomatics, 78*(6), 380.

Öst, L. G. (2008). Efficacy of the third wave of behavioral therapies: A systematic review and meta-analysis. *Behaviour Research and Therapy, 46*(3), 296-321.

Öst, L. G. (2014). The efficacy of Acceptance and Commitment Therapy: An updated systematic review and meta-analysis. *Behaviour Research and Therapy, 61*, 105-121.

Powers, M. B., Zum Vörde Sive Vörding, M. B., & Emmelkamp, P. M. G. (2009). Acceptance and Commitment Therapy: A meta-analytic review. *Psychotherapy and Psychosomatics, 78*(2), 73-80.

Ruiz, F. J. (2010). A review of Acceptance and Commitment Therapy (ACT) empirical evidence: correlational, experimental psychopathology, component and outcome studies. *International Journal of Psychology and Psychological Therapy, 10*(1), 125-162.

Ruiz, F. J. (2012). Acceptance and Commitment Therapy versus traditional Cognitive Behavioral Therapy: A systematic review and meta-analysis of current empirical evidence. *International Journal of Psychology and Psychological Therapy, 12*(2), 333-357.

Skinner, B. F. (1953). *Science and Human Behavior*. New York: Simon and Schuster.

Törneke, N. (2010). *Learning RFT: An introduction to relational frame theory and its clinical application*. Oakland, CA: New Harbinger Publications.

Kerry Beckley

6 Schema Therapy

Schema Therapy (ST) has evolved over the past 20 years to the point where it is now used both individually and with groups, with an emerging evidence-base for an increasing number of clinical presentations. It can be considered part of a broader trend in cognitive therapy which places a greater importance on information processing that is not readily available to conscious awareness (Edwards & Arntz, 2012).

Developed by Jeffrey Young, ST is primarily aimed at treating those who have entrenched interpersonal and identity difficulties associated with a diagnosis of personality disorder (Young, 1990). Individuals with more complex difficulties require the therapist to draw upon a wider range of techniques. ST combines aspects of cognitive, behavioural, psychodynamic, attachment, and gestalt models, and considers itself to be truly integrative, and continually evolving. Theoretical integration aspires to more than a simple combination of techniques, as it seeks to create an emergent theory that is more than a sum of its parts (Norcross & Halgin, 1997). Cognitive and behavioural techniques are still considered important aspects of treatment, but the model gives equal weight to emotion-focused work, experiential techniques, and the therapeutic relationship. Like cognitive behavioural therapy (CBT; see Chapter 4), it is structured, systematic, and specific, following a sequence of assessment and treatment procedures. However, the pace and emphasis on particular aspects of treatment may vary depending upon individual need.

6.1 Early Maladaptive Schemas

Young (1990) defines Early Maladaptive Schemas (EMS) as self-defeating emotional and cognitive patterns that develop early in childhood and are strengthened and elaborated throughout life. Maladaptive behaviours are thought to be driven by schemas. According to the model, schemas are dimensional, meaning that they have different levels of severity and pervasiveness. The more entrenched the schema, the greater the numbers of situations that activate it, the more intense the negative affect, and the longer it lasts. It is assumed that all individuals can relate to at least some of the schemas described in the model, although these are typically more rigid and extreme in individuals who seek psychological treatment.

Eighteen EMS are proposed in the model (see Young, Klosko, & Weishaar, 2003). By definition, they are dysfunctional and result in psychological distress. They are thought to be the result of both a child's innate temperament and early experiences, and are accumulatively strengthened through ongoing negative interactions with others. In adulthood, the person engages in a variety of cognitive, affective, and behavioural manoeuvres which enable the person to maintain, avoid, and adapt to their schemas in order to avoid experiencing overwhelming psychological distress. These coping styles take the form of Schema Surrender (giving in to the schema and accepting that the resulting negative consequences are unavoidable); Schema Avoidance (avoiding triggers internally and externally that may activate the schema); and Schema Overcompensation (acting as though the opposite of the schema was true).

6.2 Historical Origins of Schema Therapy

ST was Young's attempt to address the needs of those for whom CBT was not found to be effective. The first form of the therapy, Schema Focused Therapy (SFT), was developed in the late 1980s and can be considered an adapted form of Cognitive Therapy (CT). SFT placed a greater focus on the childhood development of schemas (or core beliefs) and the therapeutic relationship, and included experiential techniques in order to target emotional change more effectively. The key principles of SFT were the identification of schemas, their developmental origins, and the coping strategies that develop in response to the presence of schemas. Intervention in SFT was based upon an understanding of how schemas and coping strategies impacted upon the person's life and the therapeutic relationship.

By the mid-1990s, SFT was being applied to a wider range of clinical presentations, such as other personality disorders (Young & Flanagan, 1998) and eating disorders (Waller, Kennerley, & Ohanian, 2007); the model consequently evolved into Schema Mode Therapy so as to accommodate broader clinical complexity. While EMS are trait-like entities, that is, enduring features of the personality, schema modes are considered the state-like, changeable manifestations of schemas. Schema modes (see Young et al., 2003) are defined as 'self-states' that temporarily come to the fore and dominate a person's presentation, and are made up of clusters of schemas and coping strategies. In clients whose personalities are poorly integrated, schema mode states can shift rapidly from one state to another. The concept of schema modes enables therapists to work with these sudden and extreme emotional shifts more effectively. Schema Mode Therapy, now known most commonly as Schema Therapy, has become the primary model most commonly worked with today (Young et al., 2003). There can be confusion between ST and SFT, as SFT is still referred to in a number of the key research studies – although ST was the preferred term adopted by the organisation founded to provide training and certification of the model, the International Society of Schema Therapy (ISST), in 2006.

In the early 2000s, Group Schema Therapy (GST) was developed for females with Borderline Personality Disorder (Farrell, Shaw, & Webber, 2009) and male forensic patients (Beckley & Gordon, 2010). Key features of the group approach are the utilisation of group therapeutic factors (Yalom & Leszcz, 2005), the facilitators' roles as 'co-parents', and the group's capacity to engage in experiential exercises which are both schema-activating and healing for all. Unlike some practiced forms of 'group' therapy,

GST is not simply individual therapy which the rest of the group observe; the group acts as an extended family, with members who are active in the intervention for each other as well as themselves.

6.3 Key Techniques

Whilst CBT aims to teach clients to manage their negative emotions through modification of cognition, ST uses experiential techniques to evoke affect as the therapist tries to bring about change in an emotionally connected way. In the beginning of the therapy, experiential techniques such as imagery re-scripting (Arntz & Weertman, 1999) and chair-work (Kellogg, 2004) are used more frequently in order to access the person's core emotional experiences; in the later phases of therapy, there is a greater inclusion of cognitive and behavioural strategies to facilitate pattern breaking. Imagery restructuring and re-scripting are techniques commonly used in CBT for certain clinical presentations such as PTSD, Depression, and Social Phobia (Edwards, 2007; Grey, Young, & Holmes, 2002; Wild, 2009). Chair-work originates from the psychodrama work of Jacob Moreno and is a key technique in Gestalt Therapy (Perls, 1973). Therapeutic dialogues in chair-work take two forms. In 'empty chair' dialogues the person sits facing an empty chair and is asked to imagine a person in the opposite chair with whom they wish to converse. In the second form, the person moves between two chairs (or possibly more when working with modes) in order to play out an inner conflict (Kellogg, 2012). In schema therapy, this conflict is most commonly represented in schema mode dialogues. These techniques can serve as both cognitive and experiential in nature but, in ST, the focus is mainly on increasing emotional intensity, in order to increase the impact of schema healing work.

In ST, experiential techniques are used to go much deeper into unmet childhood needs and to enhance the use of the therapeutic relationship as the primary vehicle for change. It is not claimed that ST is unique in this, and there is evidence of a greater recognition of the therapeutic relationship in other broadly cognitive approaches (Gilbert & Leahy, 2007; see Chapter 10). In ST, the key relational strategies are 'Empathic Confrontation' – validating the development and continued perpetuation of schemas whilst simultaneously confronting the necessity to change – and 'Limited Re-parenting' – providing what an individual needed but did not get from their parents as children, within the boundaries of the therapy relationship. The experience of childhood is always present in the therapeutic dialogue. Even when the focus is on current issues, the aim is to understand the present in the context of the past. When the person is unclear why they are acting out in a particular way, the underlying schema or mode is traced back to its function in early life to cope with 'toxic' experiences, in order to facilitate understanding of the present.

A particular strength of ST is how easily the concepts are understood and emotionally resonate with clients. The key message is that distressing emotions in response to current issues are directly linked to early childhood experiences, and that the strategies developed in order to cope in childhood are now problematic in adulthood. It is argued that the concept of schema is more effective at conveying emotional depth as opposed to a term like "core belief", which does not capture the potency of the person's experience. Diagrammatic formulations are useful for conveying the therapist's understanding of the client, and the inclusion of images to represent the different modes can be particularly effective. Making use of such diagrams in-session can facilitate both client and therapist understanding of what is happening in the moment.

6.4 Goals of Schema Therapy

The overall aim of ST is to develop the person's Healthy Adult Mode, which is understood as fundamentally changing aspects of personality functioning. This role is modelled by the therapist in the early stages of therapy, with the therapist gradually reducing their 'active parenting' over the course of therapy as the client develops autonomy in this regard. The goals of therapy are met when the client is able to achieve the following tasks:

1. Manage the emotional impact of early unmet needs, understood as the client being able to care for their own Vulnerable Child Mode.
2. Reduce the need for maladaptive coping modes, so that the client is able to tolerate connection with their emotional world without detaching or compensating for the effect of such connection.
3. Set limits upon the expression of anger or impulsivity in order to be able to express and assert their emotional needs effectively.
4. Reduce the intensity of self-punishment and criticism as conceptualised by the Punitive or Demanding Parent Mode, so that the client becomes able to hold onto compassion for themselves and others, has permission to make mistakes, and forms realistic expectations.

6.5 The Schema Therapist

The personal qualities of the therapist are of importance in ST. A good ST therapist should not be resistant to feeling personally affected by their therapy with clients, and emphasis is placed on their capacity to maintain a limited re-parenting stance. Limited re-parenting is considered the 'heart' of ST (Farrell, Reiss, & Shaw, 2014). Therapists who are most comfortable with a structured, predictable protocol are usually not well-suited to ST. The approach requires constant adaptation and responsiveness, based on the formulation of the person whose presentation can change moment-to-moment. To create a re-parenting bond, it is vital that the therapist can be openly warm and caring – i.e., comfortable in sharing these feelings with the client. Physical touch is considered acceptable, but not essential; clearly its use needs to be carefully considered and may not be appropriate with certain clients or in specific settings. The ST therapeutic stance requires the person to have a clear understanding of their own emotional needs through the formulation of early experiences and schema development. The principle of 'complementarity', the process by which an individual's behaviour can 'pull' the other into a familiar pattern of interacting (Safran & Segal, 1990) is central. Within the ST model, this has been described as 'schema chemistry' and is understood as the interpersonal activation of schemas between individuals. This can impact on the therapist-client fit when the therapist's own schemas become activated by the interpersonal schema-driven patterns of the client. Schema chemistry is also a very useful concept in understanding the patterns of interaction which take place within mental health inpatient environments (Beckley, 2011) which is an aspect of the case study presented here.

6.6 Who Does it Work for?

ST was initially developed for treating Borderline Personality Disorder (BPD), but it is now also being used with a wider range of clinical presentations – although the evidence-base for its application outside of BPD is in its infancy. Most of the evidence thus-far has been generated for clients with BPD. Initial evidence emerged from a single-case design series, showing a significant reduction in EMS as measured on the Young Schema Questionnaire-2 (Young & Brown, 1994) and improvements in secondary outcome measures (Nordahl & Nysæter, 2005). Limitations of the study included the lack of independent evaluators and difficulties of generalising to a larger group from a single-case design.

A multi-centre trial in the Netherlands found that ST led to recovery from BPD in about half the sample, with two thirds experiencing a clinically significant improvement (Giesen-Bloo et al., 2006). ST was found to be approximately twice as effective as Transference Focused Therapy, and despite being a long term, high intensity intervention, ST was also found to be less costly and to have a much lower drop-out rate. The paper highlights the particular benefits of ST being: the transparency of the model, the re-parenting attitude of the therapist, clearly defined techniques, and the possibility to contact the therapist between sessions. A subsequent study demonstrated that ST was as effective in clinical practice as the findings in the RCT, and that the availability of telephone contact with therapists out of hours was not essential (Nadort et al., 2009).

A recent RCT demonstrated that group-based ST was an effective treatment for women with BPD (Farrell et al., 2009). Those receiving ST had lower scores on measures of BPD and higher scores on assessments of global functioning; differences were clinically significant, and sustained at six-month follow-up.

There is some evidence to suggest that ST can be useful in the treatment of Axis I disorders, particularly in the context of more complex presentations and where first-line treatments have proven unsuccessful. Ball (1998) developed Dual Focused Schema Therapy (DFST) for the treatment of substance abuse and comorbid personality disorder and evidenced its effectiveness in comparison with standard group counselling in two small-scale RCTs (Ball, 2007; Ball, Cobb-Richardson, Connolly, Bujosa, & O'Neall, 2005), although those with more severe personality disorders gained more benefit from standard group counselling. There is also an emerging body of single-case study evidence for ST across a range of clinical presentations (Bamelis, Bloo, Bernstein, & Arntz, 2012).

6.7 Criticisms of Schema Therapy

Perhaps one of the greatest limitations for ST in the UK, in the context of a resource-limited National Health Service (NHS), is the length of treatment that the approach requires. However, research is needed to establish the economic benefits of providing longer term psychological intervention for those clients who, given the nature of their enduring difficulties, often require inpatient treatment, lengthy community mental health care, or welfare support – and may come into contact with the criminal justice arena. The additional 'strain on the surroundings' (van Asselt & Bloo, 2012) in terms of informal support from family or friends is a further cost which is not well understood. Van Asselt et al (2008) were able to establish that ST was more cost-effective over a period of three years in comparison to treatment-as-usual. Studies comparing short-term psychological interventions (20 sessions or less) – which are most commonly offered to individuals with complex psychological difficulties – with longer-term therapies, such as ST, may have a greater bearing on how treatment is offered in the most cost-effective way.

James (2001) outlined some specific concerns in relation to the increasing use of ST, mainly pertaining to unskilled therapists using techniques which were outside of their range of competence, and ST being used as a panacea for a range of Axis I problems where CBT has already evinced effectiveness. There is merit in the criticism that the model can appear deceptively simple in theory, but the delivery of ST with complex challenging clients requires a high level of expertise or supervision from a certified therapist (e.g., for those embarking upon training in the model).

To summarise, schema formulation involves the establishment of patterns between early unmet needs and current difficulties, conceptualised by schemas and modes. The aim is to understand the function of current coping strategies in this context, and how they maintain the underlying schemas, and repeatedly educe emotional distress or detachment. This enables the therapist to effectively target the core unmet needs of the client, with the aim of reducing schema intensity and, consequently, the need for the coping strategies. The therapist looks for themes which persist over time and in different relational contexts to aid this process.

6.8 Formulation in Action

The case description conveys that Molly experiences a deeply-held sense of worthlessness (Defectiveness/Shame) and that she does not fit in anywhere (Social Isolation). Molly infers that social groups make her anxious and she prefers indirect forms of communication. Perhaps most poignant, is the prevalent theme that she is not valid or important to others, and that her needs do not matter (Emotional Deprivation). There is evidence of her feeling compelled to act in a compliant manner in relation to her parents (Subjugation), which suggests she is dissatisfied with her ability to assert her needs. This would be considered worthy of further exploration as the client's current relationship with her parents may be indicative of patterns of interaction established from childhood. Molly makes unfavourable comparisons with her sister, both in terms of her achievements (Failure) but also her sister being the favoured child (Defectiveness/Shame). Love and approval appear to be conditional within the family, particularly in terms of her mother.

Molly's relational template is further influenced by her observation of her parents' relationship. She portrays a significant emotional distance existing between them, with virtually all emotional interaction being supressed other than critical comments made by her mother. Molly appears to have a greater need for emotional expression than other members of the family; as a consequence of her parents' response to this, her need is experienced as a problem, and leads Molly to internalise her distress (Emotional Inhibition). Molly appears to have apportioned blame to herself for not meeting familial norms – with only fleeting evidence of her anger towards others. This would be an area for further exploration, as appropriate expression of anger appears to be an unmet need for Molly. Molly's physical complaints may relate to her frustration in not being able to communicate her emotional needs, and so they manifest as physical problems which require attention and intervention. This is linked to her sense that her emotional needs are unimportant and that physical problems are more likely to receive a response from others.

Molly's sense of herself as a problem and others as uncaring or uninterested is also evidenced in relationships outside of the family. In peer relationships, she describes herself as controlling and emotionally demanding. Further exploration would be needed to confirm the primary function of this, but her early history would suggest that this is a compensatory strategy which manoeuvres others into a position of rejecting her; likely to be reinforcing of her underlying schemas of Defectiveness/Shame and Emotional Deprivation. In ST, these schemas resulting from unmet needs represent the Vulnerable Child Mode, and they steer the direction and focus of therapy.

Molly's mother appears to be the primary attachment relationship from which the Punitive Parent Mode has developed. Love and praise were contingent on Molly behaving in ways acceptable to her mother, often with a focus on academic attainment – and other aspects of her are ignored, dismissed or actively discouraged. It would appear that Molly was partially able to manage the expectations of her mother by making herself useful, not making emotional demands, and achieving academically. However, this was achieved to the detriment of Molly's sense of personal worth – i.e., at the cost of being accepted for 'who she is' – and interaction with others created too much anxiety for her as to 'how to behave'. There is a sense that Molly's Punitive Parent Mode is very active at such times, berating her internally for being attention-seeking or a burden to others. Her father is somewhat absent in her narrative and this relationship warrants further exploration.

In adulthood, Molly's Detached Protector Mode comes to the fore when she expects to be criticised or ridiculed by others, representing a generalisation of her maternal relationship. This results in her socially and emotionally withdrawing in order to protect herself. She considers herself to be flawed and unacceptable to others, seeing herself as a "burden", and so turns down invites to social activities. This in turn results in fewer invites being made, and reinforces her underlying schemas; it is seen as evidence to support her perception that others are critical of her, and that this is pervasive across familial, social, and work relationships. There is a repeating pattern of social avoidance in response to this perception. The incident with Jack is an example of this: she feels stupid, and perceives her housemates, including Jack, to be rejecting of her, and she experiences a high level of shame. Her relationship with Danny is indicative of an underlying Abandonment/Instability schema, where the person forms intense relationships which ultimately result in them being rejected. This is worth further exploration although her account of her early experiences indicates that other (aforementioned) schemas could account for this relational pattern. It would be interesting to explore the reasons for Molly switching between avoidant and compensatory relational strategies in different contexts.

Exploration of Molly's relationship with her sister Ella may prove useful. Ella is considered the 'favoured' sister in Molly's mind, despite behaving in ways which one would assume their mother would disapprove of. Ella is one person that Molly is openly critical of, and it is possible that she is envious of Ella's apparent self-confidence and success – feeling inhibited from being able to 'please herself' in a similar way.

Molly's time in hospital parallels her early experience of family. She is accused of being dramatic and attention-seeking in her expression of distress, alienating some of the staff. Her self-harming behaviours can be understood as attempts to communicate distress and elicit support from others, but her methods of doing so result in rejection and resentment from some staff. This is a common response to behaviours understood as 'attention-seeking', often because the staff themselves feel helpless and unable to provide adequate care. Other staff are able to connect with Molly's underlying vulnerability, and so relate to her in a more empathic manner. ST would understand these differential responses in schema-mode terms, as differential connections with the modes or 'parts' of the person as if they were the 'whole' person. It is not clear which mode Molly was in when she took the overdose of pain killers. If it was an attempt to numb her emotional pain, it may represent an avoidance strategy; but, if her motivation was to seek care or attention from others, it might be better understood as an over-compensatory strategy. Certain nursing staff experienced this as a manipulation of them, rather than the behaviour being understood as a communication of Molly's genuine emotional need, and so Molly is further invalidated by her experience of in-patient treatment.

Molly's presentation at interview demonstrates very strongly the Vulnerable Child-Punitive Parent Mode interaction being played out. She initially presents in Angry Child Mode, where she is expressing her anger and distress at being ignored as she experiences it. This could be understood as evidence of a Punitiveness Schema, suggesting she sees herself and others as needing to be punished harshly for their mistakes. However, this cannot be assumed on the basis of her observed responses, as it may alternatively form part of a compensatory strategy: being critical of others as a way of receiving confirmatory criticism of herself as a response. Molly appears to revert back to self-blame very quickly and so the latter is likely to be the case.

Molly's disclosure of sexual abuse would certainly be explored further and provides further evidence that Defectiveness/Shame is likely to be a key schema. She alludes to sexual problems being far more significant than is suggested previously. This may well be a core theme in her treatment but the therapist needs to be mindful not to assume which aspects of Molly's early experience are of primary importance without careful exploration.

Molly's goals are other-directed and vague. This is not unusual and collaborative formulation would assist with some further clarification. In ST, imagery techniques would be useful to help her connect with the core unmet needs which structure and drive the therapy process. If psychiatric diagnosis was considered important to Molly, we may initially conceptualise her difficulties as Avoidant Personality Disorder (American Psychiatric Association, 2013). In terms of Axis I problems, Major Depressive Disorder may feature. However, further assessment would be required to clarify the core schemas at play, deepening the understanding of repeated patterns in different aspects of Molly's life, in order to fully appreciate the level of difficulty she may be experiencing. This is particularly important when considering whether somebody would meet the criteria for a diagnosis of personality disorder as, if the difficulties were in one domain of a person's life, this would not be an appropriate conceptualisation; that said, the information provided in the case description is adequate for developing an initial formulation from a schema perspective.

6.8.1 Schema Formulation

Molly describes a childhood characterised by fear of abandonment and rejection by others, and a sense of herself as worthless and unlovable. The family environment can be described as emotionally inhibited, which exacerbated Molly's sense that she was often in the wrong or in trouble for causing some form of irritation or inconvenience to her parents. These experiences are characterised by Defectiveness/Shame, Social Isolation/Alienation, Emotional Deprivation, and Emotional Inhibition. These Schemas are considered to represent her primary unmet needs and are conceptualised as the Vulnerable Child Mode. In response to these unmet needs it would appear that Molly may have felt anger towards others but that this anger was severely restricted in expression by the emotionally-inhibited environment and her fear of being rejected or criticised. There is a sense that her mother was the most powerful parental figure in the home, as the father is hardly mentioned – and only then in response to her mother's treatment of him. Molly may have developed a more expressive Angry Child Mode had she been in different circumstances, but instead has suppressed her emotional needs in response to the value that she sees others put upon them. This mode briefly appears on occasion. There is an absence of the Happy Child Mode in Molly's narrative; it is not clear that she has had the opportunity to experience important social and personal development opportunities that we associate with a happy childhood, and this will be an important focus in therapy.

Molly has a well-developed Punitive Parent Mode which appears frequently in her own narrative; berating her for having emotional needs, for not being stronger, and for being a burden on others. This is likely an internalised experience of her mother's treatment of Molly and there does not appear to be a protective paternal influence upon this, leaving Molly to cope with this herself.

There is evidence of Molly flipping between all three coping styles. Molly has tried hard to meet the expectations that her mother has of her – such as doing well academically, not creating a fuss, and managing her own problems – and this reflects her Compliant Surrender Mode. This mode represents Molly's attempt to feel love and approval from her mother, but appears to be ineffective. Her most prevalent coping style is one of avoidance; she quickly tends to distance herself from peers and engage in solitary hobbies or activities in order to protect herself from further criticism and rejection. There are numbing or soothing elements to some of her preferred activities, such as cleaning and the use of prescribed medication, which may function to reduce the Punitive Parent-Vulnerable Child interaction in her mind. This is best conceptualised as her Detached Protector Mode. Her goals are other-focussed and there is a likelihood that she does not have a clear sense of who she is or what she wants, indicating an underdeveloped sense of self. Molly can also act in an overcompensatory manner, being overbearing and clingy in relationships. This appears to be most likely to occur when someone has shown an initial interest in her, which she is not able to tolerate due to suggesting she is worthy of love or attention, and so she acts in ways which result in her being rejected or criticised, reaffirming the 'truth' of the underlying schemas. Her attempts to control her eating can also be understood as a compensatory strategy: as an attempt to manage her sense of defectiveness. These strategies are ineffective in meeting her emotional needs, and so Molly's sense of hopelessness and worthlessness increase and maintain her sense of self and others.

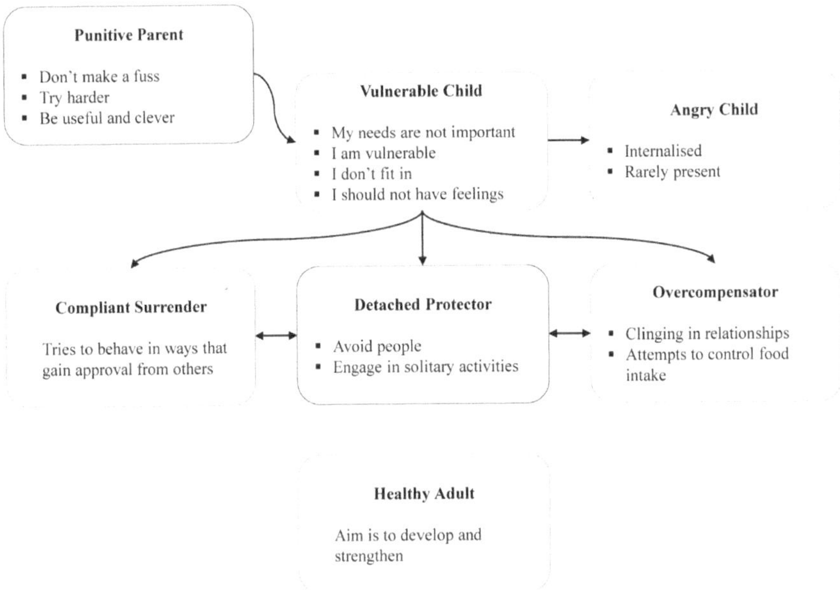

Figure 6.1: Diagrammatic Formulation

6.8.2 Intervention Objectives

Schema Therapy would begin with an extended assessment phase which would involve the use of experiential techniques in order to fully explore the links between Molly's past and current issues. The formulation is used in conjunction with these techniques as a basis for understanding how the modes interact and relate to each other. Based on the material presented, the therapist would be paying particular attention to the Vulnerable Child-Punitive Parent interaction, to increase awareness of this mode and its significant impact upon Molly's sense of self. The therapist needs to create a safe space for Molly to start to express her needs, whilst actively working on minimising the 'interruptions' of the Punitive Parent and by acting as a good parent, through praise, encouragement and validation. Molly needs to be able to connect with the therapist in this way before the other modes can actively be worked upon. Lockwood and Shaw (2012) highlight the impact of children who have been 'play-deprived' and how therapeutic play can be incorporated into experiential work to give the client permission to explore their emotions safely. Examples of how Molly could be encouraged to connect with anger include popping balloons, drawing, or a tug of war game, all of which involve permission-giving, laughter, and praise for having an emotional presence.

Once the necessary safety and trust is established, Molly can begin to explore the key childhood memories and experiences which resonate with current difficulties. Every opportunity is taken to use language and techniques which provide re-parenting interaction based on the unmet needs of the person. In Molly's case this would require a focus on the validation of her own worth and support with the expression of her needs – and for these to be listened and attended to. In imagery re-scripting, Molly would use current issues to 'track back' to their childhood origins, where there is the opportunity to replay these memories in a way which directly addresses her needs in that moment. Similarly, a focus of imagery re-scripting would be to develop and encourage Molly's Happy Child Mode, to provide repeated imagery experiences for Molly of having her needs both valued and met. Another experiential technique which may be useful with Molly would be to construct a 'no-send letter' to either/both parents in order to build her confidence in emotional expression.

The aim of this earlier phase of therapy is to build Molly's resilience and confidence, embodied by the Healthy Adult Mode. The repeated experience of experiential work aims to enable her to feel more able to deal with her current difficulties. As therapy progresses, the focus starts to shift onto the use of maladaptive coping modes in her adult life; continuing with the experiential techniques for this purpose, but also introducing cognitive and behavioural strategies to help Molly strengthen her Healthy Adult Mode outside of therapy. This can involve the use of diary cards, to track schema/mode-activating events, and the development of flashcards, to support Molly in remembering key therapy messages at times when her Vulnerable Child is most likely to be triggered. These cards could also serve as transitional objects to help Molly keep the therapist 'in mind' when the Punitive Parent Mode is active. Cognitive techniques can be useful in supporting the schema-healing process of the experiential work. Homework features in Schema Therapy but its use depends on the needs of the client. Molly could be set tasks which require her to practice expressing her needs, being assertive with her parents, and, in particular, being compassionate to herself. Depending on the goals set regarding social and relational contacts, Molly would be supported to take gradual steps towards managing her coping strategies differently and to approach feared social situations. In contrast to shorter-term therapies, this behavioural pattern-breaking work is often left until the latter part of therapy, so as not to place too many expectations on the client to have a Healthy Adult mode that is capable of such tasks. A primary therapeutic message is that change needs to be aimed at meeting Molly's needs and is not about pleasing others; helping her redistribute and re-allocate a sense of responsibility – and even blame, where appropriate – equally to other people or events in her life.

6.8.3 Challenges in Therapy

A particular difficulty which may arise is Molly's tendency to please others. Therapists are often less aware of over-compliance than they are of conflict in therapy, as it can appear as if the intervention is going well. This would be openly discussed with Molly using the formulation, and both therapist and client would be encouraged to take responsibility for noticing the Compliant Surrender mode at play. Ways to consider managing this include providing more than one option for intervention strategies, being mindful in imagery re-scripting to offer choice, and to gradually increase Molly's sense of autonomy and control over the direction of re-scripting when this is developmentally appropriate.

Molly is also likely to find it difficult to assert herself with the Punitive Parent Mode. For many clients, this mode is so intrinsic that they can find it hard to separate out the 'inner critic' from themselves. This is why experiential techniques such as chair-work can be particularly helpful, as this part of the person can be physically separated and distanced in the room. Once this has been achieved, Molly can be supported by the therapist to assert herself. It is important to distinguish this mode as originating from a critical or abusive parent, but that the mode is not *actually* the parent. Molly is likely to struggle with the concept of 'banishing' her mother, as she still has a relationship with her, and her mother is likely to have some positive influence in Molly's life. However, it is necessary for Molly to be able to more accurately apportion responsibility for her current difficulties if she is to make progress in building her Healthy Adult Mode. An important aspect of therapy would be to enable Molly to express anger or frustration. The therapist can use naturally occurring events in therapy, for example, being late or making a statement which Molly finds invalidating, to encourage Molly to express such feelings, and to experience apologies from the therapist and affirmation that her needs are important. Molly is likely to find this very difficult initially but it is important to persist with this endeavour.

6.8.4 How is Effectiveness Evidenced?

Successful intervention is ideally based on a thorough analysis of the goals set at the start of therapy. Goal attainment scaling (GAS; Kiresuk & Sherman, 1968) can be a useful to monitor emotional, behavioural, and cognitive changes over the course of therapy. There is no measure of schemas that fully incorporates their multiple elements; the YSQ-L3 (Young & Brown, 2003) is the latest version of the Young Schema Questionnaire and mainly taps into the cognitive 'core belief' aspect of schemas. Other tools include the Young Parenting Inventory (YPI; Young, 1999); Young-Rygh Avoidance Inventory (YRAI; Young & Rygh, 1994), Young Compensation Inventory (YCI; Young, 1995) and the Schema Mode Inventory (SMI; Young et al., 2007); all of which purport to measure aspects of the person's functioning in relation to the ST model. These measures are considered to complement a comprehensive clinical assessment and therefore have utility in assessing outcome. Sheffield and Waller (2012) provide a useful guide to the use of these tools in clinical practice and highlight that a reduction in scores on measures is not necessarily an indication of good clinical outcome.

In RCTs, effectiveness of particular interventions is sometimes judged on the basis of individuals no longer being considered to meet diagnostic criteria. However, diagnostic criteria and quality of life are two distinct constructs – and meaningful therapeutic benefits to quality of life may be achieved without any change in diagnostic classification. Additionally, alternative measures, such as measures of self-esteem, may complement behavioural evidence for change. Primarily it is the view of Molly – and the positive changes she makes in terms of therapy goals – that is the most valid indicator of therapeutic success. Based on the formulation, one would hope to achieve changes in Molly's ability to express and assert her emotional needs, to experience relationships with others as mutually fulfilling, and for her to experience occupational and social activities in more positive terms. Overall, from the material provided, Molly would be considered an ideal candidate for ST.

Aidan J P Hart

6.9 Schema Therapy Formulation: Critical Commentary

As I understand it, the Schema Therapy (ST) model places the origins of the client's distress within Early Maladaptive Schemas (EMS) – which are unhelpful ways of interpreting the world – and how these manifest in unhelpful ways of being in the world (maladaptive Schema Modes). EMS are themselves contingent upon negative early life experiences.

On the face of it, from a behavioural perspective, this makes sense. Early negative experiences shape up particular behaviours via direct conditioning and indirectly through rule-governed behaviour. Within such contexts, a child may learn basic avoidance-based coping. Problems arise as they get older and encounter similar situations where previously conditioned responses are now elicited in the present (e.g., via stimulus generalisation). It is likely that such behaviours will be avoidance-based (i.e. negatively reinforced) coping strategies that bring immediate relief but also delayed aversive consequences. Due to a human propensity to be more influenced by immediate over delayed consequences, the short-term avoidance is more likely to remain a part of the behavioural repertoire. This keeps the client stuck in self-defeating attempts to escape their own distress.

Whilst there are aspects of the model I can relate to, I did see what I thought were some limitations of the approach, pertaining to its inchoate evidence-base and focus on nomothetic categorisations/the concept of 'schemas'. Moreover, I found myself questioning whether 'schema' or 'schema mode' constructs are actually necessary within the approach; what do they add to the formulation?

6.9.1 Evidence-base

The approach is primarily designed for clients with a personality disorder diagnosis, with some recent attempts to apply it to other diagnoses. Considering that the approach has existed in published form for over 25 years, I was surprised at the lack of published empirical research on either outcome efficacy or theorised mechanisms of change (component analyses, for example).

I was further surprised at the lack of recognition of limitations of available outcome research. Some studies cited in the chapter had been previously reviewed by Masley, Gillanders, Simpson, and Taylor (2012) and found to be of a good standard (such as Giesen-Bloo et al, 2006). However, others (such as Farrell, Shaw, & Weber, 2009) drew more criticism; in particular, for failing to control for confounds between the ST and control (treatment as usual) groups. The lack of evidence, and the lack of recognition of limitations in the evidence-base, seemed to be a weakness.

6.9.2 Categorisation and the Concept of Schemas

Reading the chapter, I was struck by the pseudo-diagnostic categorisations and infantilising jargon ('punitive parent', 'vulnerable child') that ran through the description. EMS were discussed as if they are real and tangible things that inhabit individuals. This seemed to shift the focus onto things that people 'have' at the expense of the things that have happened to them. Explaining behaviour through schemas (which are behaviours themselves) leaves us with the added question of what is the context (i.e., an interaction with the environment) in which schemas are formed, elicited, and maintained. This surely brings us back to a focus on what has happened to the client through their lived experience of the world. Whilst ST does appear to attend to this, I am unsure what pseudo-diagnostic categorisation adds to the process. In this regard, the concept of EMS seems an unnecessary level of complication and a distraction from the variables influencing the client's distress.

Claims were made about the nature and prevalence of EMS that seemed to be unfounded and/or irrelevant to the model:

1. It is assumed that everyone to some degree has EMS. Despite the model existing in published form for over 25 years, there is no evidence that this is in fact the case and this assumption remains entirely untested and without foundation. Given

that Schema Theory originated as a model of personality disorder and research has found personality disorder to have a weighted population prevalence of 4.4% (Coid, Yang, Tryer, Roberts, & Ullrich, 2006) this seems like a fanciful claim.

2. A worrying implication of the 'everyone has schemas' assumption is that those who score minimally on a measure such as the Young Schema Questionnaire can be dismissed as being in some form of denial or protecting themselves via some form of Schema Mode. This seems to make any formulation based upon the model dangerously unfalsifiable, with no way to refute the therapist's analysis.
3. Despite the concept of EMS and Schema Modes being central to the model, there is no evidence presented as to their relation to distress. The notion that schemas drive the very behaviours we use to infer the existence of schemas seems like circular reasoning.
4. There is confusion in the model in that the shift from EMS to Modes in ST clearly suggests that EMS are not of central importance, yet EMS still form part of the definition provided for Schema Modes themselves.
5. Schemas seem unrelated or unnecessary to the formulation of distress. It is one thing to highlight a history of abandonment in significant relationships and an expectation that this will be repeated, but there is little evidence to support the notion that a person has an 'abandonment schema' residing somewhere inside them and that such a notion adds anything to treatment.
6. Whilst it is well documented that early experiences are influential in human development, the concept of EMS seems to imply that there is a mythical stage where things are set in stone. While this seems like an attractive proposition, it leaves little room for considering the impact of later events on psychological well-being and leaves the therapist to offer the unfalsifiable position that the reaction to later events is contingent upon the already identified EMS.

6.9.3 Comparison to ACT Formulation

Despite my concerns above, I was struck by the similarity in the formulations and the interventions across the two models. Both had an appropriate focus on what Molly had learned about the world and a focus on helping Molly break down ineffective patterns of avoidance. The one difference I would note would be on ACT's focus on Values and Committed Action. Whilst I could see this possibly fitting into the ST concept of the Healthy Adult Mode, the ST focus seemed to be dominated by avoidance goals (thinking and feeling less about the bad stuff) rather than appetitive goals (having more of what is wanted). Whilst the merits of either approach remain an empirical question, I was left wondering what happens when a client is in Healthy Adult Mode: does therapy focus on helping the client to grow further, or is it assumed that the client will do this for themselves now that they are a healthy adult and no longer in need of a therapeutic parent figure?

6.9.4 Final Thoughts

I could relate to many aspects of the ST formulation and treatment plan – recognising evident parallels with my own (ACT-based) formulation of Molly. However, what struck me most about the ST formulation was that there seemed to be a lack of obvious or necessary connection to the concept of schemas (either in the form of EMS or Schema Modes).

The question I was ultimately left with was: In order to be effective, does schema therapy really need schemas at all?

Kerry Beckley

6.10 Author Response

The reviewer suggests there is a lack of evidence for theorised mechanisms of Schema Therapy. There is evidence for components of Schema Therapy, in terms of schemas and modes, but it was not possible to include a thorough review within the confines of a formulation chapter. It is accepted that there are methodological weaknesses in the available research but, overall, this does not detract from the positive body of evidence which is accumulating for Schema Therapy.

The reviewer suggests that the concepts of schemas and modes are 'infantilising'. It is not my clinical experience that either clients or professionals experience them this way, and the concepts provide a framework for developing a narrative that is often underdeveloped in clients with 'toxic' and traumatic early attachment experiences. Schemas and modes are in no way 'pseudo diagnostic': modes in particular are terms that are developed in collaboration with the client to ensure personal resonance – to represent these as distinct categories would be to misuse the model.

The reviewer appears to be suggesting that Schema Therapy considers the presence of schemas as evidence of personality disorder. Schemas are considered to be trait-like constructs that develop from unmet needs, and which help us to consider the function of peoples' actions. Development of schemas is not considered to be 'disorder'-specific: such consideration would detract from the goal of reducing an 'us and them' distinction from individuals who already feel isolated or different from others. A schema therapist does not formulate from the results of a psychometric tool in isolation, and the suggestion that this is the case indicates a misunderstanding on the part of the reviewer. The reviewer also appears to have confused the concepts of schema and core belief in suggesting that there is no evidence linking schemas with distress; schemas have an inherent emotional component, which is activated alongside the cognitive, physical, and visual elements.

The model confusion alluded to in schemas and modes is a valid criticism and therapists less familiar with the model can sometimes underestimate the importance of the thematic underpinnings of a person's mode state, which results in the techniques having less clarity in application. However, there is no mythical stage where schemas are 'set' just as there is no mythical stage when behavioural patterns become ingrained. Like other therapies, Schema Therapy aims to increase clients' insight into their difficulties and applies a particular framework to guide movement towards therapeutic change: using the therapy relationship to develop a relational template that enables clients to interact with others in ways which results in their core needs being met. How we as therapists achieve this will forever be a source of debate, and the research repeatedly tells us that the key to achieving it is the quality of the therapeutic relationship. If formulations using apparently disparate psychological models can agree on the primary issues of the client, perhaps the differences in approach are somewhat irrelevant in delivering psychological therapy?

References

American Psychiatric Association. (2013). *Diagnostic and statistical manual of mental disorders* (5th ed.). Arlington, VA: American Psychiatric Publishing.

Arntz, A., & Weertman, A. (1999). Treatment of childhood memories: Theory and practice. *Behaviour Research and Therapy, 37*(8), 715-740.

Ball, S. A. (1998). Manualized treatment for substance abusers with personality disorders: Dual focus schema therapy. *Addictive Behaviors, 23*(6), 883-891.

Ball, S. A. (2007). Comparing individual therapies for personality disordered opioid dependent patients. *Journal of Personality Disorders, 21*(3), 305-321.

Ball, S. A., Cobb-Richardson, P., Connolly, A. J., Bujosa, C. T., & O'Neall, T. W. (2005). Substance abuse and personality disorders in homeless drop-in center clients: symptom severity and psychotherapy retention in a randomized clinical trial. *Comprehensive Psychiatry, 46*(5), 371-379.

Bamelis, L., Bloo, J., Bernstein, D., & Arntz, A. (2012). Effectiveness studies. In M. van Vreeswijk, J. Broersen & M. Nardort (Eds.), *The Wiley-Blackwell handbook of schema therapy: Theory, research, and practice* (pp. 585-598). Chichester: John Wiley & Sons.

Beckley, K. (2011). Making sense of interpersonal dynamics: A schema focused approach. In P. Willmot & N. Gordon (Eds.), *Working positively with personality disorder in secure settings: A practitioner's perspective* (pp. 172-187): John Wiley & Sons.

Beckley, K., & Gordon, N. (2010). Schema therapy within a high secure setting. In A. Tennant & K. Howells (Eds.), *Using time, not doing time: Practitioner perspectives on personality disorder and risk* (pp. 95-110). Chichester: Wiley Blackwell & Sons.

Edwards, D. (2007). Restructuring implicational meaning through memory-based imagery: Some historical notes. *Journal of Behavior Therapy and Experimental Psychiatry, 28*(4), 306-316.

Edwards, D., & Arntz, A. (2012). Schema therapy in historical perspective. In M. van Vreeswijk, J. Broersen & M. Nardort (Eds.), *The Wiley-Blackwell handbook of schema therapy: Theory, research, and practice* (pp. 3-26). Chichester: John Wiley & Sons.

Farrell, J. M., Reiss, N., & Shaw, I. A. (2014). *The schema therapy clinician's guide: A complete resource for building and delivering individual, group and integrated schema mode treatment programs*. Chichester: John Wiley & Sons.

Farrell, J. M., Shaw, I. A., & Webber, M. A. (2009). A schema-focused approach to group psychotherapy for outpatients with borderline personality disorder: A randomized controlled trial. *Journal of Behavior Therapy and Experimental Psychiatry, 40*(2), 317-328.

Giesen-Bloo, J., Van Dyck, R., Spinhoven, P., Van Tilburg, W., Dirksen, C., Van Asselt, T., . . . Arntz, A. (2006). Outpatient psychotherapy for borderline personality disorder: Randomized trial of schema-focused therapy vs transference-focused psychotherapy. *Archives of General Psychiatry, 63*(6), 649-658.

Gilbert, P., & Leahy, R. L. (2007). *The therapeutic relationship in the cognitive behavioral psychotherapies*. London: Routledge.

Grey, N., Young, K., & Holmes, E. (2002). Cognitive restructuring within reliving: A treatment for peritraumatic emotional 'hotspots' in posttraumatic stress disorder. *Behavioural and Cognitive Psychotherapy, 30*(1), 37-56.

James, I. A. (2001). Schema therapy: The next generation, but should it carry a health warning? *Behavioural and Cognitive Psychotherapy, 29*(4), 401-407.

Kellogg, S. (2012). Using chairwork dialogues in schema therapy. In M. van Vreeswijk, J. Broersen & M. Nardort (Eds.), *The Wiley-Blackwell handbook of schema therapy: Theory, research, and practice* (pp. 197-207). Chichester: John Wiley & Sons.

Kellogg, S. H. (2004). Dialogical encounters: Contemporary perspectives on "chairwork" in psychotherapy. *Psychotherapy: Theory, Research, Practice, Training, 41*(3), 310-320.

Kiresuk, T. J., & Sherman, M. R. E. (1968). Goal attainment scaling: A general method for evaluating comprehensive community mental health programs. *Community Mental Health Journal, 4*(6), 443-453.

Lockwood, G., & Shaw, I. (2012). Schema therapy and the role of joy and play. In M. van Vreeswijk, J. Broersen & M. Nardort (Eds.), *The Wiley-Blackwell handbook of schema therapy: Theory, research, and practice* (pp. 209-227). Chichester: John Wiley & Sons.

Nadort, M., Arntz, A., Smit, J. H., Giesen-Bloo, J., Eikelenboom, M., Spinhoven, P., . . . van Dyck, R. (2009). Implementation of outpatient schema therapy for borderline personality disorder with versus without crisis support by the therapist outside office hours: A randomized trial. *Behaviour Research and Therapy, 47*(11), 961-973.

Norcross, J. C., & Halgin, R. P. (1997). Integrative approaches to psychotherapy supervision. In C. E. Watkins (Ed.), *Handbook of psychotherapy supervision* (pp. 203-222). Hoboken, NJ: John Wiley & Sons.

Nordahl, H. M., & Nysæter, T. E. (2005). Schema therapy for patients with borderline personality disorder: A single case series. *Journal of Behavior Therapy and Experimental Psychiatry, 36*(3), 254-264.

Perls, F. S. (1973). *The gestalt approach & eye witness to therapy*. Palo Alto, CA: Science & Behavior Books.

Safran, J., & Segal, Z. V. (1990). *Interpersonal process in cognitive therapy*. New York: Basic Books.

Sheffield, A., & Waller, G. (2012). Clinical use of schema inventories. In M. van Vreeswijk, J. Broersen & M. Nardort (Eds.), *The Wiley-Blackwell handbook of schema therapy: Theory, research, and practice* (pp. 111-124). Chichester: John Wiley & Sons.

van Asselt, A. D. I., Dirksen, C. D., Arntz, A., Giesen-Bloo, J. H., Van Dyck, R., Spinhoven, P., . . . Severens, J. L. (2008). Out-patient psychotherapy for borderline personality disorder: cost-effectiveness of schema-focused therapy v. transference-focused psychotherapy. *The British Journal of Psychiatry, 192*(6), 450-457.

van Asselt, T., & Bloo, J. (2012). Cost-effectiveness of schema therapy. In M. van Vreeswijk, J. Broersen & M. Nardort (Eds.), *The Wiley-Blackwell handbook of schema therapy: Theory, research, and practice* (pp. 585-598). Chichester: John Wiley & Sons.

Waller, G., Kennerley, H., & Ohanian, V. (2007). Schema-focused cognitive behavioural therapy for eating disorders. In L. P. Riso, P. L. du Toit, D. J. Stein & J. E. Young (Eds.), *Cognitive schemas and core beliefs in psychological problems: A scientist-practitioner guide* (pp. 139-175). Washington, DC: American Psychological Association.

Wild, J. (2009). Imagery and the self in social phobia. In L. Stopa (Ed.), *Imagery and the threatened self: Perspectives on mental imagery and the self in cognitive therapy* (pp. 94-111). New York: Routledge.

Yalom, I. D., & Leszcz, M. (2005). The theory and practice of group psychotherapy. New York: Basic Books.

Young, J. E. (1990). *Cognitive therapy for personality disorder: A schema focused approach.* Sarasota, FL: Professional Resource Exchange Inc.

Young, J. E. (1995). *Young Compensation Inventory.* New York: Cognitive Therapy Center of New York.

Young, J. E. (1999). *Young Parenting Inventory.* New York: Cognitive Therapy Center of New York.

Young, J. E., Arntz, A., Atkinson, T., Lobestael, J., Weishar, M. E., van Vreswijk, M. F., & Klokman, J. (2007). *The Schema Mode Inventory (SMI).* New York: Schema Therapy Institute.

Young, J. E., & Brown, G. (1994). Young Schema Questionnaire (second edition). In J. E. Young (Ed.), *Cognitive therapy for personality disorders: A schema focused approach* (Rev. ed., pp. 63-76). Sarasota, FL: Professional Resource Exchange.

Young, J. E., & Brown, G. (2003). *Young Schema Questionnaire–long form, third edition (YSQ-L3).* New York: Schema Therapy Institute.

Young, J. E., & Flanagan, C. (1998). Schema-focused therapy for narcissistic patients. In E. F. Ronningstam (Ed.), *Disorders of narcissism: Diagnostic, clinical, and empirical implications* (pp. 239-268). Washington, DC: American Psychiatric Press.

Young, J. E., Klosko, J. S., & Weishaar, M. E. (2003). *Schema therapy: A practitioner's guide.* New York: Guilford Press.

Young, J. E., & Rygh, J. (1994). *Young-Rygh avoidance inventory.* New York: Cognitive Therapy Center of New York.

Thomas Schröder, Angela Cooper & Rohan Naidoo

7 Intensive Short-term Dynamic Psychotherapy (ISTDP)

Intensive Short-term Dynamic Psychotherapy (ISTDP) is one of a group of modern psychodynamic therapies that have been developed over the past 50 years. While firmly rooted in psychoanalytic theory, they are briefer than analytic treatments and require a more active stance from the therapist. ISTDP is closer to the instrumental[3] than the relational[4] view of therapy and nearer the intrapsychic than the interpersonal end of the spectrum.

Like other dynamic psychotherapies, ISTDP is based on the understanding that a patient's presenting difficulties are adaptations to anxiety or psychic pain caused by intrapsychic conflicts (Coughlin Della Selva, 2004; Frederickson, 2013; Ten Have-De Labije & Neborsky, 2012). It is *experiential*, in that half of the therapeutic task is to contact the patient's conflicted emotions as *here-and-now bodily experiences*, the second half being cognitive insight into how avoiding such experiences was the root cause of the patient's difficulties (Davanloo, 1990; Malan, 2000). The approach, developed by Davanloo (Davanloo, 1990, 2001, 2005), is based on Freudian theory, but applied through a set of techniques he claims remove the problems of therapeutic resistance. Malan (1980) suggests that ISTDP is the most significant step forward in psychodynamic psychotherapy since Freud, concluding that "Freud discovered the unconscious; Davanloo has discovered how to use it therapeutically" (p.23).

Put simply, intrapsychic conflicts are defined as defences against painful hidden feelings, which evoke anxiety[5] when approaching conscious awareness (Malan, 1979). Within ISTDP, 'hidden feelings' are summarised as the mixed emotions arising towards a caregiver when the attachment bond is ruptured: initial love and connection give way to protest and rage, then guilt about the rage, then grief and deep sadness about the loss of love.

Thus, the person is conflicted: one part of them wishes to contact and work through these anxiety-provoking attachment emotions, another acts to suppress them. The fundamental therapeutic task is to encourage the former as the path to therapeutic change, and help the patient disown the latter – the cognitive-behavioural patterns perpetuating their difficulties. It is a process of pressing toward emotion,

3 The notion that personal change occurs through specific techniques delivered on the basis of a good therapeutic relationship.

4 The notion that personal change occurs through a good therapeutic relationship delivered via the medium of specific techniques.

5 This utilises Freud's second theory of anxiety, where forbidden feelings and wishes stimulate a rise in anxiety; such anxiety acting as a signal for defences to be activated, which ward off the 'dangerous' emotions, and thus dampen anxiety (Erwin, 2002)

regulating the anxiety evoked, and blocking the maladaptive defences that hinder this process, summarised by Malan's triangle of conflict, which the Triangle of Person explains was formed in the past, and repeated in the patient's current life, as well as in the here-and-now of their relationship with their therapist (see Fig. 7.1, adapted from Malan, 1979).

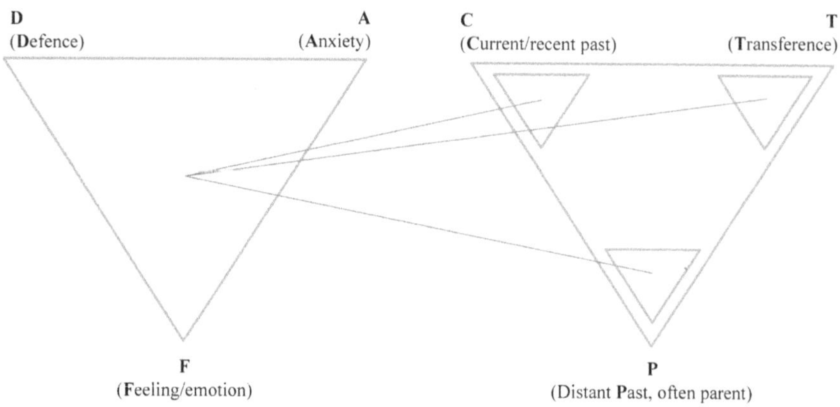

Figure 7.1: Left: Triangle of Conflict, illustrating the conflict between defence, anxiety, and hidden feeling. Right: Triangle of Person, illustrating that conflicts formed in the distant past generalise to current or recent and transference relations

A hallmark of ISTDP is the precision with which emotions, anxiety, and defence are operationalised and worked with (Coughlin Della Selva, 2004). For an emotion to be experienced, it must be:
- labelled (e.g., guilt),
- felt as a physical sensation (e.g., sinking heavy feeling in chest/upper stomach), and
- its impulse explored in fantasy (acting to put the situation right).

Full experience often precipitates the next attachment emotion (e.g., anger leads to guilt, guilt to sadness, sadness to love).

Anxiety signals that such emotions are surfacing; and this experience is diagnostic of how quickly painful feelings can be worked through. If the therapist observes striated muscle activity, this signals that the patient can bear the emotions being activated, giving a 'green light' for further pressure. Smooth muscle activity or cognitive-perceptual disruption suggest easing off pressure toward feelings as this may be too anxiety-provoking for the patient (see Tab. 7.1).

Table 7.1: Pathways of anxiety (adapted from Coughlin Della Selva, 2004)

Striated Muscle Anxiety	Smooth Muscle Anxiety	Cognitive-Perceptual Disruption
Hand clenching	Bladder urgency	Drifting, dissociation, confusion
Tension in arms, neck, shoulders, and head	Gastrointestinal – IBS	Visual blurring/narrowing of visual field.
Sighing respiration	Vascular – migraine headache	Fainting, freezing, fugue states
Abdomen, legs, feet tense, and fidgeting	Bronchi – asthma	Hallucinations
	Localised or generalised pain	
	Auto-immune disorders	

Defences may be either tactical ways of avoiding interpersonal contact with the therapist, or more formal character structures (Coughlin Della Selva, 2004; Frederickson, 2013), as summarised in Table 7.2.

Table 7.2: Types of defence (adapted from Coughlin Della Selva, 2004)

Tactical Defences		Formal (Character) Defences	
Non-verbal	**Verbal**	**Repressive**	**Regressive**
Avoiding eye contact	Vagueness	Intellectualisation	Projection
Arms and legs crossed	Diversification	Rationalisation	Denial
Smiling and laughing	Sarcasm	Minimisation	Dissociation
Weepiness	Argumentative	Displacement	Acting out
Temper tantrums	Contradictory	Reaction formation	Somatisation
	Rate of speech		

Davanloo conceptualised the Central Dynamic Sequence (discussed further below) as a systematic method for how, in an idealised therapeutic scenario, the therapist can help the patient overcome their defensive processes in order to contact their hidden attachment emotions (Tab. 7.3, adapted from Abbass, Town, & Driessen, 2013; Davanloo, 1990, 2001, 2005).

Table 7.3: The Central Dynamic Sequence (adapted from Davanloo, 2001)

1	**Inquiry** Asking about client's inner emotional difficulties, history of the difficulties, severity, significant life events, goals; establish will to explore emotions.
2	**Establish triangle of person** Focus on a specific example of when these difficulties were experienced; either in current life, transference relationship, or in past.

Table 7.3: The Central Dynamic Sequence (adapted from Davanloo, 2001) (continued)

3	**Working triangle of conflict** Encourage client's experience of feelings, block or restructure defences that prevent feelings from rising, regulate anxiety into striated pathway. Level of intensity rises to pressure, challenge, and head-on-collision as necessary.
4	**Breakthrough** Unconscious therapeutic alliance and patient's desire to experience emotions in transference, current, or past, overcomes the defensive parts of psyche that avoid emotion and perpetuate difficulties.
5	**De-repression** As the unconscious is unlocked, there is a de-repression of freely associated memories, meanings, and images that have dynamic significance.
6	**Interpretation** Cognitive linking together of de-repressed material into a coherent more conflict-free narrative, that better makes sense of the client's internal world. Focus on linking the triangle of person and conflict to build new insights.

7.1 Historical Origins

Davanloo's method, built on over 40 years of analysing videotaped sessions (Abbass et al., 2013), is immersed in Freudian theory, addressing the unconscious and feared 'taboo' emotions towards attachment figures, thus also owing a great debt to Attachment Theory (Bowlby, 1989). It echoes with the short-term, body-oriented work of Alexander and French (1946), Ferenczi and Rank (1925) and Gestalt therapy (Smith, 1976), and builds upon the short-term approach of Davanloo's mentor, Peter Sifneos (1987). David Malan has been instrumental in the history of short-term dynamic psychotherapies, and since the late 70s has been a great advocate for ISTDP (Gustafson, 1986). Now, Davanloo's work has inspired a broader range of Experiential Dynamic Therapies, in which many of his former students have blended his approach with their own. Examples include Accelerated Empathic Therapy (Fosha, 1992), Affect Phobia Therapy (McCullough et al., 2003), Experiential Short-Term Dynamic Therapy (Osimo, 2003), and Attachment-Based ISTDP (Ten Have-De Labije & Neborsky, 2012).

7.2 Unique Features

A first-time observer of ISTDP would see a number of distinctive features. Practically, there is an initial 2-3 hour 'trial therapy' session in which the therapist concentrates on intervention and assesses the patient's response. Research indicates this as the best way to assess suitability for treatment (Gustafson, 1987), with factors such as diagnosis or severity of trauma having little predictive value. It is also likely that sessions are videotaped, for the therapist to review and reflect on. Qualitatively, there is an unerring, moment-by-moment focus on the patient's inner world – aspects which seek true expression and experience ranged against those parts that wish to hide from and avoid such deep contact with the 'true self.' The therapist's interventions are highly active and at first glance confrontative, as 'minimum respect' is shown to the defences that inhibit the patient's true self and perpetuate their suffering (Davanloo, 1990). Furthermore, attention is paid not just to the 'conscious alliance' of patient and therapist, but signals from the 'unconscious alliance' – such as the manner in which the patient delivers their words, double meanings, gestures, body language, signals of anxiety, physical symptoms etc. – that give the therapist clues to unconscious emotions (Davanloo, 1990, 2001). Altogether, the observer may begin to see how ISTDP is distinctive by blending elements from other approaches into a range of interventions that cohere around Davanloo's (2005) 'metapsychology of the unconscious'. Although this is underpinned by Freudian principles, Malan (2010) notes a sharp distinction between ISTDP and traditional analysis:

> "Instead of allowing the client's defences to operate and then offering interpretations at a time when the client is receptive, an ISTDP practitioner seeks to help the client confront and disown their defences as they are activated, facilitating the here-and-now experiencing of the emotions which they repress."

This difference, he reflects, is justified by the finding that defences are less impenetrable, and the therapeutic relationship far stronger, than first thought.

7.3 Empirical Evidence

The empirical base for ISTDP is still developing. Abbass, Town, and Driessen's (2013) review found 21 outcome studies pertaining to personality disorders, somatic disorders, depression and anxiety disorders, and mixed samples that reference Davanloo's method in their description of treatment. Of these studies, 13 (including 5 RCTs), met criteria for meta-analysis and used common outcome measurements. Effect sizes (Cohen's *d*) ranged from 0.84 for interpersonal problems to 1.51 for depression, and for the 5 studies with follow-up data (general psychopathology and interpersonal problems), these effects were maintained at follow-up ranging from six months to ten years. More widely, a 2014 Cochrane Review (Abbass et al., 2014), updating an earlier review (Abbass, Hancock, Henderson, & Kisely, 2006), included 33 studies of short-term psychodynamic psychotherapy (STPP) for 2173 randomised participants with common mental health disorders, in which problems with emotional regulation were purported to play a causative role. Across general, somatic, anxiety, and depressive symptoms (plus interpersonal problems and social adjustment), there was significantly greater improvement in the short and medium term (with the exception of somatic symptoms in the short-term) relative to controls. Although effect sizes increased at long-term follow-up, some effects did not attain statistical significance. More specifically, post-hoc tests revealed that effect sizes were significantly greater for those studies using Malan/Davanloo's approach than other STPP methodologies. However, given the heterogeneity of samples, study types, and methodological limitations of the original research, the authors advise caution when interpreting these promising results.

7.4 Critiques and limitations of ISTDP

Despite the above, empirical support for ISTDP is still limited. Although Davanloo's techniques have evolved to include more 'fragile' patient populations (Abbass et al., 2013; Whittemore, 1996), it is not recommended for those with poor impulse control or with active psychotic symptoms. However, suitability is largely judged on response to the initial trial therapy session. As an emotionally challenging approach, ISTDP demands great ability to tolerate intense emotion from both therapist and patient, and, for the therapist, awareness of counter-transference (Abbass, 2004). There is a danger of using specific ISTDP techniques without sufficient understanding, training, and supervision. To press on feelings when the patient is too anxious, or using regressive defences, can increase suffering. Applying specific factors too frequently, without paying sufficient attention to common factors, can also lead to misalliances (McCarthy, 2009). Furthermore, without reflective capacity, the abuse of therapist-patient power differentials and the devaluation/idealisation of the model or the therapist are potential risks; indeed, Gustafson (1986) caricatures Davanloo's approach as akin to 'revelatory religious experience' – the 'saviour therapist' offering the promise of transformative experience to the suffering patient. More broadly, debate about the validity and utility of psychoanalytic thought remains; however, this is now modified by new evidence in the field of neuroscience (Johnston & Malabou, 2013). Nevertheless, there is sound evidence for ISTDP's efficacy, consistent with trans-theoretical models, suggesting that intense emotional experience and cognitive re-appraisal are both necessary for therapeutic change (Ecker, Ticic, & Hulley, 2012).

7.5 Formulation in Action

The chronological narrative of Molly's history and current predicament meshes well with the developmental perspective of a psychodynamic theoretical frame. The account appears much more structured then the story that a client would normally tell, but, reading through it, our mental process is similar to that of listening during an assessment – organising and reorganising material as it emerges, noticing gaps and ruptures in the narrative, and trying to get empathic access to her experience while monitoring our emotional reactions.

Starting with her current circumstances, the first thing we notice is Molly's relative dearth of intimate relationships (single, lives alone, one close friend whom she talks to once a week on the phone, use of social media, solitary hobbies). Her feelings towards her parents make us wonder whether she generally protects herself against demands she perceives as excessive (and might feel guilty about not being able to meet) by avoiding close contact. This leads to an initial dynamic hypothesis about withdrawal as an adaptation to (defence against) the anxiety arising from a conflict between a wish (to be close) and a feared reaction (to be taken advantage of). This preliminary understanding will be modified in light of subsequent information.

In considering her early personal history, we wonder about Molly's ambivalent feelings about her sister Ella. It must be difficult for her, due to her agonising conflict between love and anger, to feel reliant on someone of whom she is jealous, possibly envious. When she allows herself to do so, she fears she might be unable to contain her aggressive impulses and end up hurting someone she loves. Here we notice that our emotional engagement changes – something of her distress arrives in us, possibly helped by the direct quotes. Now we need to ask ourselves whether her experience resonates with our own. Having excluded that potential cause for our reaction, we are left with the hypothesis that we have been invited into a complementary countertransference, providing in our minds something that meets Molly's internal need.

Continuing, it seems that Molly learned a model of intimate relationships from her parents: where getting too close can be destructive and hostile feelings are best expressed at a distance. In their effort to modulate aggression, they may have controlled affection too, leading them to perceive Molly as overly emotional, and Molly experiencing home life as lacking warmth. We also would assume that her emotional demands might have stirred up her parents' mixed feelings, who would have defended themselves against their own ambivalence towards intimacy, first through criticism – to express their rage – and then guilty withdrawal to protect Molly from the consequences of their feelings. We also find ourselves speculating that Molly perceived an absence of unconditional acceptance from her parents, notably her mother. Maybe the best way she could secure love and attention was by being a self-reliant high achiever, and could only safely express her dependency needs when being physically unwell. Having little confidence that others would give her freely what she needed, being controlling and demanding would appear a reasonable – and sometimes successful – strategy.

From the account of her early adulthood it appears that Molly's adaptation of high achievement initially worked well, but that she developed another adaptation – social withdrawal – to cope with the anxieties about mixed feelings created by exposure to others. It is not clear why this might be so, but an initial hypothesis would be that she can easily feel shamed; maybe something resonates with her experience of mother's disappointed looks. As being prone to shame is often linked with high self-criticism, we now wonder about early interpersonal experiences of being criticised that she may have taken on board. The intrusion on her sexual encounter with Jack would have served to sensitise her further to shame – because of her engaging in self-attack rather than healthy anger to express her hurt about the incident – and may have evoked her conflict regarding the potential destructiveness of intimate contact. It is possible that, when feeling vulnerable, she tried the familiar strategy of being demanding and controlling but was unsuccessful with Jack. This would have triggered more hurt and reactive anger about Jack's unavailability, leading to further self-attack and shame. This maladaptive process reinforces the idea that others shame her, rather than her shaming herself, recreating an old pattern we imagine to have originated in intimate moments with her parents. This would serve to further strengthen her embarrassment and fear of being ridiculed, to the point where social withdrawal appeared the only possible coping strategy.

The account of Molly's adulthood shows her adaptation of high achieving becoming less productive (working as a classroom assistant rather than a teacher) and increasingly undermined by her interpersonal withdrawal. In the relationship with Danny, her propensity for being seen as controlling and demanding now becomes clearer as a defence against the abandonment anxiety arising from a conflict between her wish to be close and special and her experience of being rejected, leading to intense mixed feelings toward him. As before, this unhelpful adaptation brings about the feared consequence, leading to her taking an overdose. We would understand this as a desperate attempt to avoid recognising her murderous feelings towards Danny by turning them against herself, in a final effort to protect the attachment.

So far, we notice two gaps in Molly's narrative: The absence of her father and the lack of any expression of rage. Maybe her idealisation of Danny links to her early experience of father not having fulfilled his required role of being desirable but containing the desire – either by being absent or by not providing safe boundaries. Ella seems the one person whom Molly feels safe to argue with. In her absence, she is turning her hostility towards herself, leading to her hospitalisation. The ward staff's split attitudes towards her possibly reflect her abandonment conflict – they either react against her frantic efforts to belong, or relate to her loneliness.

Molly's time with her parents, after being discharged from hospital, clarifies her use of achievement to secure parental approval. This can now be understood as an adaptation (reaction formation) to the anxiety arising from her anger at excessive demands, both from others and from herself. It serves her well for a time, allowing her to succeed at work and be content at home, but breaks down in the face of interpersonal conflict, possibly mirroring the dynamic between herself and Ella.

Molly's initial attempts to resolve her problems – replacing interpersonal contact with internal dialogue and trying to control her appetites – are unsuccessful. Her childhood success in eliciting care from the family doctor possibly facilitates seeking help from her current GP, resulting in her referral for psychological therapy.

The initial consultation shows an unexpected readiness to move towards change. She appears emotionally engaged, willing to express anger (at her therapist, her parents, and herself), and openly demonstrates her conflict between wanting to be needy and self-reliant at the same time. It is possible that she uses her defence of high achieving (being a good patient) to cope with her anxiety about being looked at critically by the therapist. We expect that subsequent sessions with an ISTDP therapist would stimulate her defence of withdrawal.

The important disclosures in the subsequent sessions confirm and sharpen up the preliminary hypotheses. The experience of sexual abuse would have confirmed her sense that being close to someone makes her vulnerable to being exploited and hurt, possibly exacerbating her sense of intimacy as being potentially destructive, and reminding her of her own destructive feelings towards others that need to be kept locked down at all costs.

At this point we can think of two conflict formulations, each relating to an aspect of Molly's current predicament:

1. Her desire to be close and taken care of, which is activated when others are getting close to her, is in conflict with her experience of being taken advantage of. She protects herself and others against the anxiety-provoking feelings consequent to being hurt in the past by withdrawal or acting out.
2. Her wish to be special to another is in conflict with her experience of being critically evaluated and conditionally loved. She protects herself and others from the intense mixed feelings connected to previous rejections by striving hard to achieve. When she fails in this, she protects herself and others even further against the rage about her needs not being met, by trying harder to please and, when this fails, by turning her anger against herself.
3. We can see how her repeated adaptive reactions have developed into a 'character defence' – a habitual way of responding to perceived threats (see Table 7.2). It is maintained by 'cyclical maladaptive patterns' (Strupp & Binder, 1984), where her expectations of others lead her to dysfunctional interpersonal interactions that serve to confirm and strengthen her negative expectations. We would expect these patterns to be enacted with her therapist.

7.5.1 Initial Formulation Diagram

Our initial formulation is diagrammatically represented in Figure 7.2. It serves as a preliminary guide to intervention, as shown in the right-hand column, but will be updated and modified as we observe how Molly reacts in sessions.

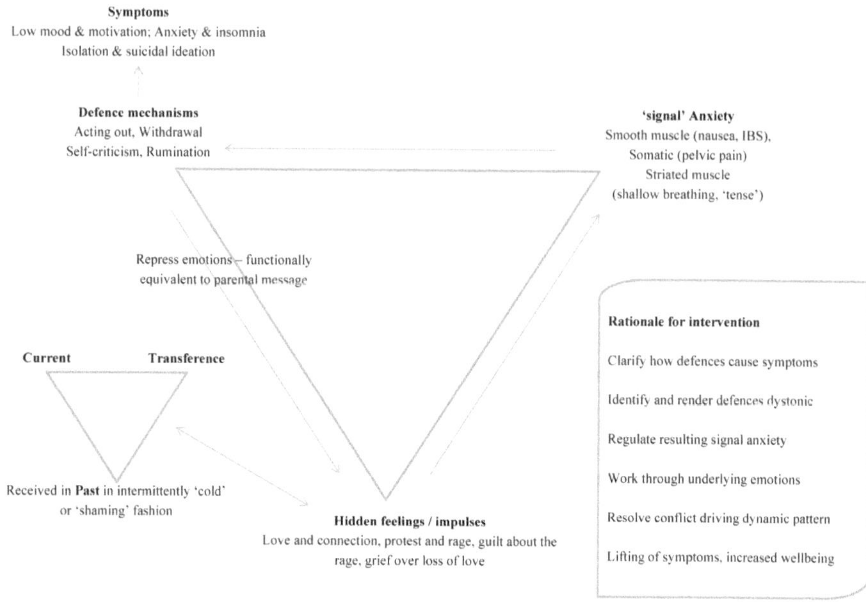

Figure 7.2: Initial formulation

7.5.2 Intervention Objectives

From an ISTDP perspective, we understand that the patient's symptoms and presenting problems are the inevitable result of excessive reliance on defences against anxiety-provoking feelings. While these defences often had an adaptive function in the past, their automatic and habitual use undermines the patient's current functioning. Without awareness of the feelings triggering the anxiety and driving the defences, the patient is 'driving blind' and is no longer making conscious choices. Therefore, the therapeutic task involves helping patients face and experience, rather than avoid, their conflictual feelings about the present and the past, as rapidly as possible and to the greatest degree that they can bear (Davanloo, 1990). Davanloo's research suggests that the visceral experience of anxiety-provoking feelings, in the here and now, serves as a trigger, *unlocking the unconscious*6 and revealing the core of the patient's conflicts (Davanloo, 1990, 2001, 2005). In this way, the unresolved feelings from the past become clear and are available for re-evaluation. Patient and therapist can then

6 Theoretical concepts specific to Davanloo's ISTDP (1990, 2001, 2005) will be italicised from here on to distinguish them from any colloquial meaning. Definitions of key concepts are provided as a glossary in Table 7.4

discover the true nature of the underlying cause of the patient's distress and resolve it at the source. Once these conflicts are consciously understood and their relationship to the patient's symptoms and suffering clarified, a process of working through and resolution of the presenting problems can take place. During this process, it is essential that patients gain insight into their own inner dynamics – in particular, the ways in which their inner conflicts (Triangle of Conflict; Fig. 7.1) are repeated in their interpersonal relationships (Triangle of Person; Fig. 7.1).

The interventions used in ISTDP are designed to create in-session mobilisation of emotional processes that lead to a rise in *complex transference feelings* (CTF). The specific mechanisms that lead to this rise are thought to be the simultaneous increases in *treatment resistance*, *unconscious anxiety*, *therapeutic alliance*, and the experience of feelings (Davanloo, 2005; Johansson, Town, & Abbass, 2014). Taken together, these mechanisms represent the unique approach of ISTDP and, importantly, its theoretical roots directly underpin them; they have been empirically validated and have been found to maximise therapeutic effectiveness. A patient's rise in CTF indicates that a painful unconscious conflict can be brought to the surface. Our job as therapists is to identify and intensify this conflict in order to get to the buried feelings underneath. The feelings being mobilised (CTF), together with the therapeutic alliance, represent one of two key forces seen to be fundamental in accessing unresolved attachment emotions; Davanloo (1987) termed this the *Unconscious Therapeutic Alliance* (UTA). The UTA is the healing force within the patient that wants to obtain emotional freedom and brings forth important dynamic information that both the patient and therapist can use to get to the core emotional conflicts driving the problems. However, as the UTA and CTF rise, there is an opposing force termed *Unconscious Resistance*, which is triggered by unconscious anxiety. This can be understood as any unconscious defence that operates in the therapy relationship to keep painful, attachment based, anxiety-provoking feelings out of awareness. If this force remains, it begins to *resist* the therapeutic task and prolong the patient's suffering. Therefore, a key part of this approach is to actively weaken the resistance in order to allow the attachment-based feelings to rise, leading to an *unlocking of the unconscious*.

7.5.3 Potential Problems

In order to assess the unique problems that each patient seeks help for, a *psychodiagnostic evaluation* is undertaken. This *dynamic* process is guided by the patient's response to each therapeutic intervention, and highlights the feelings that the patient is in conflict with, their unconscious anxiety channels, the defences that create the symptoms, and the patient's self-observing capacity (Frederickson, 2013). Based on the severity of response across these domains, Davanloo (1990, 2005) defined two spectra of patients suitable for ISTDP. The first is called the *Spectrum of Psychoneurotic Disorders* and the second is the *Spectrum of Fragility* (see Fig. 7.3).

The position on the spectra indicates the ease with which a breakthrough to the unconscious can be achieved and the different types of interventions that may be required (e.g. *pressure, challenge, head-on collision, and/or cognitive recapitulation*). Davanloo (1990, 2005) observed through his empirical research a strong relationship between a patient's attachment traumas, the intensity of reactive pain, rage, guilt about the rage, and their patterns of anxiety and resistance. In essence, the greater the magnitude of these conflicted feelings, the more severe the anxiety, and the more entrenched the defences to avoid experiencing these feelings (Abbass et al., 2013). Those placed on the first spectrum tend to have had less severe attachment trauma, yet display more treatment resistance due to their ability to defend against feelings. They have more access to striated anxiety, and use more mature defences such as repression. Those placed on the latter spectrum tend to have had more insecure attachments, making it harder for them to defend against their feelings, so their anxiety becomes dysregulated and is often channelled into non-striated pathways, with the use of more primitive defences such as acting out.

It is only following a detailed psychodiagnosis that the nature of the therapeutic task can be fully realised, and the core elements of the treatment process tailored, to ensure the therapeutic objectives are achieved as efficiently and effectively as possible.

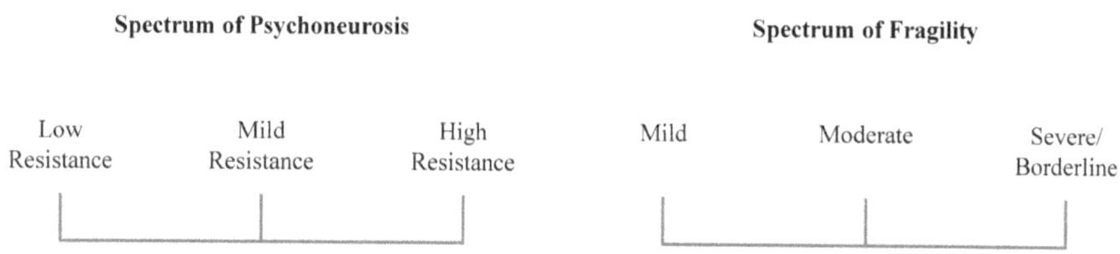

Figure 7.3: Spectra of Psychoneurosis and Fragility (Adapted from Abbass, Town, & Driessen, 2013)

7.5.4 Indicators for the Achievement of Intervention Objective

Put simply, ISTDP aims to replace symptoms and pathological defences with healthier adaptations that benefit the patient (Malan & Coughlin Della Selva, 2007). In order to achieve this, Davanloo outlined the Central Dynamic Sequence, which, broadly speaking, is designed to create an intrapsychic crisis where the dominance of the patient's healing forces over those of the resistance leads to an *unlocking of the unconscious*. During an *unlocking*, the patient experiences intense complex feelings towards the therapist or other current figure. This experience is linked to feelings towards past figures and emotion-laden memories about painful feelings, situations, and events from the past, such as adverse childhood experiences. At this point, clear links, memories and images associated with core attachment and other related traumas become accessible (Town, Abbass, & Bernier, 2013). During this process, unconscious anxiety and defences are significantly reduced in favour of emotional awareness and processing, enabling the working through and healing of previously unresolved emotions in a new, healthy, and mature way (Davanloo, 1980). One may surmise that the event of *unlocking of the unconscious* sets the stage for psychotherapeutic change during ISTDP, and recent research suggests this to be the case (Johansson et al., 2014; Town et al., 2013).

7.5.5 Effectiveness

Davanloo (1990) stated that he believed the therapeutic effects found within ISTDP were "uniquely effective" and that those effects were produced by "specific rather than non-specific factors". As discussed, the effectiveness of ISTDP is determined by the patient's response to the specific interventions employed throughout the Central Dynamic Sequence. This sequence has been empirically associated with persistently effective outcomes across a range of disorders (Abbass et al., 2013; Davanloo, 2005). Immediate changes are often most noticeable in the *unlocking* and the *working through* stages, with longer term change found in follow-up interviews over months and years (Abbass, 2002a, 2002b; Coughlin Della Selva, 2006; Davanloo, 1990).

During these stages, key processes associated with change are observed, including: de-repression of memories, experiencing and gaining insight into painful emotions, and consciously modulating feelings. These outcomes are thought to weaken unconscious associations and connections, and have been consistently associated with measures of physical and emotional health (Coughlin Della Selva, 2004; Town et al., 2013). As patients become more conscious of their feelings and behaviours, without undue anxiety or defensive processes getting in the way, there is an increase in psychological flexibility and the opportunity for adaptive choices to be made. This, in turn, makes way for major therapeutic benefit, including: symptom relief, character change, improved relationships, and emotional freedom. Coughlin Della Selva (2004, p. 171) highlighted that the depth and stability of any changes are put to the test when a patient faces a conflictual situation and demonstrates the following:

a. reduced anxiety
b. reduced reliance on defensive processes
c. increased emotional activation and affective expression
d. cognitive and emotional insights into the relationship between the Triangle of Conflict and the Triangle of Person
e. a sense of hope and mastery that overrides feelings of helplessness
f. increased adaptive capacity indicating psychological growth

As the original problems the patient sought help for are resolved, these outcomes can be observed as occurring automatically in response to situations inside and outside of therapy. When this happens, it suggests that transformational change has been achieved, whereby new learning has replaced old implicit associations, leading to deep, profound, and lasting change (Ecker et al., 2012).

7.5.6 Practical Interventions

The initial phases of Molly's ISTDP assessment would involve establishing an intrapsychic focus and enquiring into the nature of the problems she is experiencing. Gaining an internal focus is crucial; without it no psychotherapy can take place. The enquiry phase would consider, in detail, the most recent precipitant to Molly's problems, as this is likely to generate important information regarding the nature of her inner conflicts (Malan & Coughlin Della Selva, 2007). From the outset, the therapist is active and creates an atmosphere of emotional engagement, which constitutes the start of the phase of *pressure* (Davanloo, 1990).

Pressure is a series of tailored interventions that serve to bring the visceral experience of feelings, patterns of defences, and/or anxiety to light (Abbass, Joffres, & Ogrodniczuk, 2008). In the early stages, we put *pressure* on the patient to be specific, to examine their internal world, and to engage with the therapist in this endeavour. Doing so activates the attachment system and thus each area of the Triangle of Conflict. As signals of unconscious anxiety or defence emerge, they are carefully assessed and this determines how the therapist should proceed; if Molly responds with striated anxiety we examine the defences she has been using and link these defences to her presenting problems. We help her see how her defences have been hurting her and encourage her to relinquish them in order to *unlock* her true feelings. If Molly responds in ways that indicate fragility in her character structure, our interventions would focus on building her ego adaptive capacity by oscillating the interventions of *pressure* and *cognitive recapitulation*. This process is designed to bring multidimensional psychic and cognitive integration, as well as structural changes, so that Molly's capacity to withstand her unconscious anxiety and the painful feelings underneath is increased before any *unlocking* can take place (Davanloo, 1990, 2005).

7.5.7 Techniques

In order to identify what technical interventions one might need to apply, the first major task is to determine Molly's discharge pattern of anxiety. As we have not had the opportunity to assess Molly's response to intervention, we are not able to undertake an accurate *psychodiagnostic evaluation*. However, for the purposes of this chapter, we can consider the information we have been given and speculate how we might proceed.

Molly has been complaining of nausea and has a recent diagnosis of idiopathic pelvic pain and Irritable Bowel Syndrome (IBS); in response to situations at work, Molly has also reported experiencing 'butterflies' in her stomach and needing the toilet more often. These functional and somatic symptoms can indicate a pattern of unconscious anxiety that is channelled into the smooth muscles (Abbass, 2005). We also have evidence that instead of experiencing feelings, Molly tends to either act out or internalise them, for instance by taking an overdose of painkillers, becoming tearful when discussing her situation at work, expressing anger through confrontation, criticism, temper tantrums, and internalising anger through heavy self-criticism and self-blame. These defences would be considered regressive and self-punishing. We are also made aware of several interpersonal interactions, which have culminated in the unhelpful and maladaptive response of withdrawal. Collectively, this information suggests that Molly's presentation is complex, with low tolerance across a number of domains, including: anxiety tolerance, emotional tolerance, and tolerance for emotional closeness and intimacy.

Consequently, a stepwise approach is indicated, and this would be applied through the graded format of ISTDP (Coughlin Della Selva, 2006). In the graded format, cycles of *pressure* (1) are followed by a rise in *CTF* and *Unconscious Anxiety* (2). When the anxiety approaches the threshold beyond *striated*, *pressure* is reduced and *recapitulation* of the process is performed (see Fig. 7.4).

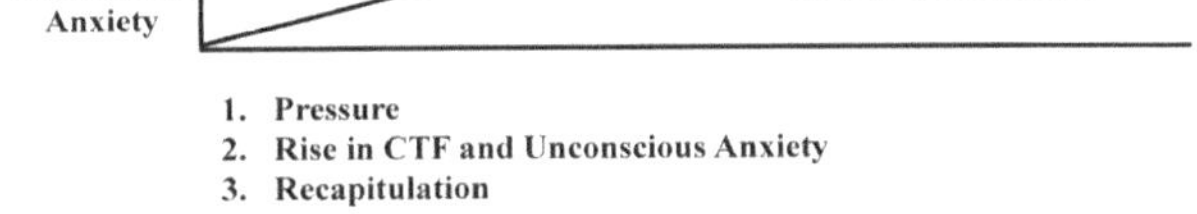

Figure 7.4: The graded format of ISTDP (adapted from Abbass & Bechard, 2007)

As soon as anxiety returns to a tolerable state (striated zone), gentle *pressure* is applied again; whenever anxiety is too high, "depressurizing" techniques are employed once more (Coughlin Della Selva, 2004). Each round should involve a slight increase in intensity, thus building, in a graded fashion, Molly's ability to tolerate her anxiety, feelings, and impulses directly. Consolidating insights into her internal dynamics is achieved by repeated cognitive analysis of the process. Once Molly's discharge pathway of anxiety has fully shifted to the striated muscle system, higher levels of *pressure* and challenge as per the standard format of ISTDP can be applied (Davanloo, 1990). The process of recapitulation reduces regressive processes, creates more mature defences, and thus "changes character" (Abbass & Bechard, 2007, p. 18). If this systematic analysis is not done, Davanloo (1990) notes that defences can re-establish themselves and symptom reduction is slower.

7.5.8 Fit of Techniques With Theoretical Approach, Formulation, and Intervention Objectives

Molly's unique adaptations to her past emotional environment are described through the Triangle of Conflict, with specific reference to the type of anxiety and defences she presents with; this then guides our intervention efforts. The technical interventions used, based on attachment and psychodynamic theory, are designed to stimulate the attachment system in order to get to the root of her presenting problems. The interventions of *pressure* and *recapitulation* are tailored to preparing the way for Molly to be able to tolerate the intensity of her unconscious feelings and the core conflicts that have been driving her suffering. As Molly begins to understand her feelings are reactive to interpersonal situations, she will see how her unresolved feelings towards others in the current and past are being enacted time and time again, in an automatic and unconscious fashion. As her unconscious is exposed to rage, and guilt about the rage, due to the overt and covert traumas of emotional coldness, dismissal, and criticism, she will then be able to experience the pain and grief about these situations and the losses they represent. Working through these reactive emotional stages should give way to previously forbidden feelings of love, longing, and connection that are at the core of the attachment system. As this process is repeated, and more of Molly's unconscious is brought into conscious awareness, her brain will begin to create autobiographical coherence, and in doing so, enable her to resolve her inner conflicts now, as an adult, with all of her current capacity.

Once Molly understands her key conflicts around closeness and intimacy, and how she has been defending herself from these, she will have the opportunity for new adaptive choices that align with her true values and her true self. This process should clear the way for her to experience major therapeutic benefit across multiple domains of functioning.

In summary, our initial formulation is a starting point for making sense of Molly's predicament. Much of the important information that will help us and her to a better understanding will emerge over the course of therapy, in response to interventions that are grounded in psychodynamic theory, but also guided by close observation of her moment-to-moment reaction.

Table 7.4: Glossary of key terms

Term	Definition	Examples
Central Dynamic Sequence	Empirically derived series of therapeutic processes as described in Table 7.3	N/A
Cognitive Recapitulation	Clarifying statement often used to reduce *pressure* and build capacity by cognitively linking emotions, anxiety and defence in the here and now.	"So we can see that when you just spoke about your anger, you turned it inwards onto you and then you experienced stomach cramps. Is this where your anger goes?"
Complex Transference Feelings	Combination of mixed feelings simultaneously experienced towards the therapist, which link to unresolved emotions about past attachment traumas.	Mixed feelings towards the therapist include: positive appreciation and irritation. Unresolved emotions from the past include: love, pain, rage, guilt and grief.
Treatment Resistance	Any (often unconscious) defence that operates to block and resist: the experience of mixed feelings emotional closeness with the therapist the therapeutic endeavour	Passivity, ambivalence, compliance, defiance, detachment, denial.
Pressure	Focused efforts to encourage the patient to emotionally engage with themselves and with the therapist.	"What emotion are you experiencing right now in your body? "How do you feel towards me when I ask you that question?"
Challenge	Once the patient can see their defences, they are encouraged to not use them and to face their feelings instead	"Now that you're aware of detaching from me, yet your body is taking some deep sighs, could we look at the feelings coming up towards me if you don't detach?"
Head-on-collision	Clarification and challenge of treatment resistant defences with an emphasis on the consequences of the defence and an encouragement to overcome it collaboratively.	"Now that you can see how denying your true experience prevents us from getting to know what you really feel and stops me from helping you, can we have a look at the emotions you are having right now so we can face reality together, otherwise you continue to remain alone with these experiences?"

Table 7.4: Glossary of key terms (continued)

Unlocking of the unconscious	The psychic state in which a patient's healthy desire to heal and reveal their hidden thoughts, feelings and impulses overcomes the part that wants to keep them stuck and suffering.	N/A
Working through	A process of making cognitive and experiential links, building conscious narratives and amplifying the therapeutic process.	"So now we can see that the anger you had towards me was linked to intense rage and guilt towards your Father who hurt you by leaving the family home. These feelings led to a deep sense of grief and a longing to be close to him again, all of which is very painful to process, but it has been driving your avoidance of intimate relationships now and leading to your loneliness and anxiety about closeness. Can you see that, too?"

Anna Tickle & Michael Rennoldson

7.6 ISTDP Formulation: Critical Commentary

We approach this critique of the ISTDP formulation from a systemic position. The systemic assumptions we draw upon include:

- Therapeutic practice is enhanced when it adopts a 'circular' understanding of causation.
- Attention needs to be paid to the social, economic, and cultural context of clients.
- The role of formulation, or hypothesising, is principally to catalyse change in a system, rather than accurately describe the origins of psychological distress.
- Therapists should pay particular attention to the potential hazards of their work, and avoid inadvertently contributing to oppressive practice.

Our critique highlights general points of overlap and difference between ISTDP and systemic practice. At first glance the two respective conceptual systems (or at least the language used to describe them) are very different. We are struck in particular by the mechanical aspects of the ISTDP view of the psychosocial world, as well as by its confident use of the language of dysfunction. Metaphors from the physical world abound: anxiety is assessed for its 'striation'; 'pressure' is applied until particular thresholds are crossed; repressed feelings are 'unlocked'. Whilst these ideas undoubtedly have utility for some clients, we also anticipate potential hazards arising from this mechanical viewpoint. We would consider this one amongst many ways of describing the social and psychological worlds with no special claim to truth.

Formulation within systemic practice focuses on the present and the social context of the person, whereas ISTDP is concerned with a person's intrapsychic world and its origins in early relationships. However, there are also points of connection. Both approaches draw upon the insights of attachment theory to bridge the social and intrapsychic worlds. Both also appear to hold recurring patterns of relationships as being of central importance in the difficulties that bring clients to therapy.

7.6.1 Formulation Content

The two conflict formulations highlight apparently repeating patterns in Molly's relationships. However, on closer reading we found little 'circularity', in the sense of explaining the contribution and interaction of all parts of a system. Instead the formulations focus on *Molly's* behaviour, feelings, and indeed 'failures' of the strategies she has tried to use. It could be argued that the 'success' or 'failure' of strategies can only arise in the context of particular responses by others.

Assuming the causation of Molly's problems lies in early parental and sibling relationships is highly linear, and risks what might be described as a teleological error. Molly's life is read as the almost inevitable playing out of early unconscious conflict. This risks neglecting the contribution of more recent or current contexts and failing to account for exceptions to the problem. For example, within the formulation, the experience of sexual abuse is interpreted as confirming or exacerbating a pre-existing conflict. However, it seems equally plausible that sexual abuse might have been completely at odds with Molly's previous experience, shattering her assumptive world (Janoff-Bulman, 1985). From a systemic perspective, the placement of causation in early relationships seems arbitrary.

The intrapsychic location of difficulties could have some benefits for some clients. It could offer Molly a sense that change is within her reach and control, as opposed to relying on others who may not buy into the process of therapeutic change. That said, it would have to be balanced against the potential for Molly to feel blamed for her difficulties. There may also be broader risks of using therapy only to reduce the distress and change the individual behaviour of victims of sexual abuse, rather than also addressing social aspects such as acknowledgement, accountability, and justice.

More broadly, the ISTDP formulation pays little attention to Molly's social and cultural context. This reflects the limited information available in the case material, but is probably also a product of the intense focus upon Molly's intrapsychic experience. For example the putative self-protective function of striving hard to achieve, identified in the second conflict formulation, may have equally significant meaning in Molly's experience of gender, social class, education, and family history.

7.6.2 Role of Formulation

The impression given is that formulation plays a relatively modest role in directing the therapy. More important are the technical assessments and procedures of the therapy, which rely on information gleaned from the client's behaviour within the therapy room. This is a similarity with a systemic approach. Both favour the use of therapeutic technique according to therapist judgement within the session, rather than following a sequence of interventions that could be mandated by a formulation. However, there are clear differences too. Within a systemic approach, formulation ideas may be discussed 'as if' they are true, but their real purpose is to stimulate change within a system. It would concern us if an ISTDP formulation is intended to be treated as a set of truthful propositions about what is really going on for a person. This raises questions of what follows for the client if the formulation turns out to be false, and what degree of confidence we can have in the ontology and discovery procedures underpinning ISTDP.

7.6.3 Client Experience

The question of how clients experience ISTDP seems not to have been addressed within research. What can be easily found online if querying the client experience of ISTDP is an article from VICE magazine that suggests the experience 'has a weird edge to it, like a psychological fight club run out of a church basement' (Keefe, 2013). The confrontational approach aims to create change within sessions at the time when the individual's defences are 'activated'. This has some similarity to the use of 'enactment' within structural family therapy, in which the therapist allows the family to engage in spontaneous transactions and then suggests alternatives (Minuchin & Fishman, 1981). Allowing therapists to use confrontational techniques whilst maintaining a belief in their own privileged access to the truth of a person's life might risk at least a poor experience of therapy, if not adverse outcomes (Masson, 1988). Family therapy has not always taken this sufficiently seriously (Reimers & Treacher, 1995), we hope the ISTDP community will.

Thomas Schröder, Angela Cooper & Rohan Naidoo

7.7 Author Response

The 'systemic' assumptions guiding this commentary are rather commonplace: Sure, context is important, formulations need to be action-oriented, therapists should avoid being oppressive, and circular understandings often help (though they do not necessarily enhance practice). All this is fairly unremarkable; the commentary's misunderstandings are far more informative: Mistaking 'striated anxiety' for a metaphor, rather than a description of the neurophysiology of emotion, points to one of the defining features of ISTDP (and by implication to one of the shortcomings of the systemic view) that we may not have sufficiently emphasised in our chapter – like other psychodynamic approaches it is an embodied therapy. From Freud's model of psychosexual stages, empathising with the infant's somatic experience (see Mitchell, 1974), via Reich's 'character armour' and Winnicott's 'psycho-somatic integration', to modern trauma therapy, the visceral aspects of experiencing have continually been privileged over the verbal/cognitive ones. Insight, however cleverly constructed and contextually aware, is held to be useless without its emotional and physical substrate. The client's moment-to-moment sensory experience, rather than any mechanical view of intrapsychic structures, is the ISTDP therapist's guide to intervention. In this sense, clearly "the 'success' or 'failure' of strategies can only arise in the context of particular responses by others", as the commentary postulates.

Another misunderstanding concerns circularity. The systemic position's aversion to linear accounts is strangely at odds with its emphasis on narrative. The Aristotelian structure of a story having a beginning, a middle, and a (preliminary) end makes intuitive sense to many clients; it directly meshes with their experience of life and may give them hope that their own future storylines can be rewritten from the position they are currently inhabiting. On that basis, circular formulations, such as 'repetition compulsion', 'cyclical psychodynamics' (Wachtel, 2014), or 'active phantasies' (Symington, 1984), then help to make sense of interpersonal maintenance cycles – the very opposite of a "teleological error", assuming an "inevitable playing out of early unconscious conflict". The client's encounter with the therapist constitutes the setting where such circular patterns can be experienced directly – rather than intellectually apprehended – and potentially modified or replaced.

A similar misapprehension relates to the role of formulations. Whether based on Malan triangles or on developmental sequences, ISTDP formulations are working hypotheses that have to be modified, revised, substantially changed, or even discarded in light of each individual client's reactions. Such understandings are of necessity specific, transitory, and incomplete. Their validity is supported or challenged by the client's physical and emotional response, rather than by their fit with a preconceived blueprint. Yes, theory is important, though primarily by helping therapists to keep their bearings and continue thinking while under pressure.

Finally, we are firmly in agreement with the need to obtain accounts of clients' experiences of ISTDP from sources other than therapists' case studies. Good qualitative research is indeed required to provide these, so that we are not taken in by a journalist's second-hand pastiche masquerading as an authentic client voice, such as the one rendered by Keefe (2013), referred to above.

Acknowledgement: The authors wish to thank Dr Patricia Coughlin Della Selva for her comments on a draft of the manuscript.

References

Abbass, A. A. (2002a). Intensive short-term dynamic psychotherapy in a private psychiatric office. *American Journal of Psychotherapy, 56*(2), 225-232.

Abbass, A. A. (2002b). Office based research in intensive short-term dynamic psychotherapy (ISTDP): Data from the first 6 years of practice. *Ad Hoc Bulletin of Short-Term Dynamic Psychotherapy, 6*(2), 5-13.

Abbass, A. A. (2004). Idealization and devaluation as barriers to psychotherapy learning. *Ad Hoc Bulletin of Short-Term Dynamic Psychotherapy, 8*(3).

Abbass, A. A. (2005). Somatization: Diagnosing it sooner through emotion-focused interviewing. *Journal of Family Practice, 54*(3), 231-239.

Abbass, A. A., & Bechard, D. (2007). Bringing character changes with Davanloo's intensive short-term dynamic psychotherapy. *Ad Hoc Bulletin of Short-Term Dynamic Psychotherapy: Practice and Theory, 11*, 26-40.

Abbass, A. A., Hancock, J. T., Henderson, J., & Kisely, S. (2006). Short-term psychodynamic psychotherapies for common mental disorders. *Cochrane Database of Systematic Reviews.*

Abbass, A. A., Joffres, M. R., & Ogrodniczuk, J. S. (2008). A naturalistic study of intensive short-term dynamic psychotherapy trial therapy. *Brief Treatment and Crisis Intervention, 8*(2), 164-170.

Abbass, A. A., Kisely, S. R., Town, J. M., Leichsenring, F., Driessen, E., De Maat, S., . . . Rusalovska, S. (2014). Short-term psychodynamic psychotherapies for common mental disorders. *The Cochrane Library.*

Abbass, A. A., Town, J. M., & Driessen, E. (2013). Intensive Short-Term Dynamic Psychotherapy: A Review of the Treatment Method and Empirical Basis. *Research in Psychotherapy: Psychopathology, Process and Outcome, 16*(1), 6-15.

Alexander, F., & French, T. M. (1946). *Psychoanalytic Therapy: Principles and Application.* New York: Ronald Press.

Bowlby, J. (1989). *The making and breaking of affectional bonds.* Abingdon: Routledge.

Coughlin Della Selva, P. (2004). *Intensive Short-Term Dynamic Psychotherapy: Theory and technique.* London: Karnac Books.

Coughlin Della Selva, P. (2006). Emotional processing in the treatment of psychosomatic disorders. *Journal of Clinical Psychology, 62*(5), 539-550.

Davanloo, H. (1980). *Short-term dynamic psychotherapy.* New York: Jason Aronson.

Davanloo, H. (1987). Unconscious therapeutic alliance. In P. Buirski (Ed.), *Frontiers of Dynamic Psychotherapy* (pp. 64-88). New York: Mazel and Brunner.

Davanloo, H. (1990). *Unlocking the unconscious: Selected papers of Habib Davenloo.* Chichester: Wiley.

Davanloo, H. (2001). *Intensive short-term dynamic psychotherapy: selected papers of Habib Davanloo.* Chichester: John Wiley & Sons Inc.

Davanloo, H. (2005). Intensive short-term dynamic psychotherapy. In B. J. Sadock & V. A. Sadock (Eds.), *Kaplan and Sadock's Comprehensive Textbook of Psychiatry.* US: Lippincott Williams & Wilkins.

Ecker, B., Ticic, R., & Hulley, L. (2012). *Unlocking the emotional brain: Eliminating symptoms at their roots using memory reconsolidation.* London: Routledge.

Erwin, E. (2002). *The Freud encyclopedia: Theory, therapy, and culture.* New York: Routledge.

Ferenczi, S., & Rank, O. (1925). *The development of psychoanalysis.* Washington, DC: Nervous and Mental Disease Publishing Company.

Fosha, D. (1992). *Accelerated Empathic Therapy (AET): History, development and theory.* London: John Wiley & Sons.

Frederickson, J. (2013). *Co-creating change: Effective dynamic therapy techniques*. Kansas City: Seven Leaves Press.
Gustafson, J. P. (1986). *The complex secret of brief psychotherapy*. New York: Norton.
Janoff-Bulman, R. (1985). The aftermath of victimization: Rebuilding shattered assumptions. In C. R. Figley (Ed.), *Trauma and its wake: The study and treatment of posttraumatic stress disorder*. (Vol. 1, pp. 15-35). Bristol: Brunner/Mazel.
Johansson, R., Town, J. M., & Abbass, A. (2014). Davanloo's Intensive Short-Term Dynamic Psychotherapy in a tertiary psychotherapy service: overall effectiveness and association between unlocking the unconscious and outcome. *PeerJ, 2*, 1-20.
Johnston, A., & Malabou, C. (2013). *Self and emotional life: Philosophy, psychoanalysis, and neuroscience*. New York: Columbia University Press.
Keefe, S. (2013, November 23). The controversial therapy that deliberately enrages patients. *VICE*. Retrieved from: http://www.vice.com/en_uk/read/this-controversial-therapy-tries-to-piss-people-off-on-purpose
Malan, D. H. (1979). *Individual psychotherapy and the science of psychodynamics*. London: Butterworths.
Malan, D. H. (1980). The most important development in psychotherapy since the discovery of the unconscious. In H. Davanloo (Ed.), *Short-term dynamic psychotherapy*, (pp. 13-23). Northvale, NJ: Aronson.
Malan, D. H. (2000). Beyond Interpretation: Initial Evaluation and Technique in Short-Term Dynamic Psychotherapy. Part II. *International Journal of Intensive Short-Term Dynamic Psychotherapy, 14*(4), 83-106.
Malan, D. H. (2010). *Introduction to ISTDP. Keynote Address*. Paper presented at the The third oxford conference on experiential dynamic therapy, St. John's College, Oxford, UK.
Malan, D. H., & Coughlin Della Selva, P. (2007). *Lives transformed: A revolutionary method of dynamic psychotherapy*. London: Karnac Books.
Masson, J. M. (1988). *Against therapy*. Monroe, ME: Common Courage Press.
McCarthy, K. S. (2009). Specific, common, and unintended factors in psychotherapy: Descriptive and correlational approaches to what creates change. *Publicly accessible Penn Dissertations*, 62.
McCullough, L., Kuhn, N., Andrews, S., Kaplan, A., Wolf, J., & Lanza Hurley, C. (2003). *Treating Affect Phobia: A Manual for Short-term Dynamic Psychotherapy*. New York: Guilford Press.
Minuchin, S., & Fishman, H. C. (1981). *Family therapy techniques*. Cambridge, MA: Harvard University Press.
Mitchell, J. (1974). *Psychoanalysis and feminism*. London: Allen Lane.
Osimo, F. (2003). *Experiential short-term dynamic psychotherapy: A manual*. Bloomington: Authorhouse.
Reimers, S., & Treacher, A. (1995). *Introducing user-friendly family therapy*. Hove: Psychology Press.
Sifneos, P. E. (1987). *Short-term dynamic psychotherapy: Evaluation and technique*. New York: Springer.
Smith, E. W. (1976). *The growing edge of Gestalt therapy*. Michigan: Brunner/Mazel.
Strupp, H. H., & Binder, J. L. (1984). *Psychotherapy in a New Key: A Guide to Time-limited Dynamic Psychotherapy*. New York: Perseus.
Symington, N. (1984). Phantasy effects that which it represents. *The International journal of psychoanalysis, 66*, 349-357.
Ten Have-De Labije, J., & Neborsky, R. J. (2012). *Mastering intensive short-term dynamic psychotherapy: a roadmap to the unconscious*. London: Karnac Books.
Town, J. M., Abbass, A., & Bernier, D. (2013). Effectiveness and cost effectiveness of Davanloo's intensive short-term dynamic psychotherapy: does unlocking the unconscious make a difference? *American Journal of Psychotherapy, 67*(1), 89-108.

Wachtel, P. (2014). *Cyclical psychodynamics and the contextual self: The inner world, the intimate world, and the world of culture and society*. New York: Routledge.

Whittemore, J. W. (1996). Paving the Royal Road: An Overview of Conceptual and Technical Features in the Graded Format of Davanloo's Intensive Short-Term Dynamic Psychotherapy. *International Journal of Short-Term Psychotherapy, 11*(1), 21-39.

Anna Tickle and Michael Rennoldson

8 Systemic Family Therapy

Systemic family therapy has evolved across geographical locations since the early 1950s. Clinically, it developed in the context of a number of therapeutic movements, including child guidance clinics, marriage counselling, and sex therapy. Whilst it is theoretically rooted in the interdisciplinary field of systems theory, or cybernetics, systemic family therapy has prided itself upon its development from practice to theory. It has also been open to influence from a heterogeneous range of other psychotherapeutic approaches and wider intellectual currents. Distinct phases of development are often identified, within which more specific schools have emerged, frequently connected with specific practitioners or clinics. These are outlined in detail elsewhere (e.g., Dallos & Draper, 2010). We present a brief overview of some of these schools before focusing on an integration of enduring systemic ideas that characterises contemporary systemic practice, especially in the UK (Vetere & Dallos, 2003). We use 'systemic family therapy', 'family therapy', and 'systemic practice' interchangeably to refer to therapeutic practice based upon systemic principles; other therapies delivered to family groups based upon different theoretical principles (for example behavioural family therapy; Falloon, 1988) are not discussed here.

Key systemic approaches include:

- *Structural family therapy*, largely developed by Salvador Minuchin (e.g., 1974) and colleagues in New York in the late 1950s and 1960s.
- *Strategic family therapy*, developed initially during the late 1960s and 1970s at the Mental Research Institute (MRI) in Palo Alto, California. Key figures included Don Jackson, John Weakland, and Paul Watzlawick (e.g., Watzlawick, Weakland, & Fisch, 1974). Strategic approaches were further developed during the late 1970s and 1980s in Milan by a group including Mara Selvini Palazzoli, Luigi Boscolo, Gianfranco Cecchin, and Guiliana Prata (e.g., Selvini Palazzoli, Boscolo, Cecchin, & Prata, 1980). Later, the group divided and 'post-Milan' approaches were developed (e.g., Cecchin, 1987).
- *Social constructionist approaches* began to influence systemic therapy from the late 1980s onwards. This influence is particularly evident in narrative therapy, developed in the 1990s by Michael White from Australia and David Epston from New Zealand.
- *Solution Focused Brief Therapy* also sits within systemic approaches. It was developed during the 1980s by Steve de Shazer, Insoo Kim Berg, and colleagues in the Milwaukee Brief Family Therapy Centre.

8.1 The Central Tenets of Systemic Family Therapy

8.1.1 Systems Theory

The interdisciplinary study of systems theory (Von Bertalanffy, 1950) underpins family therapy. It is this theoretical framework, alongside an emphasis upon working with several people at once, that distinguishes family therapy from other therapeutic approaches. Systems theory assumes that the behaviour of a system can only be understood by considering the individual characteristics of elements within the system, *and* the relationship between these elements. Families are 'systems' of people, which in turn relate to wider social systems. As individual experience is seen as fundamentally interpersonal, rather than intrapersonal (Vetere & Dallos, 2003), psychological distress is viewed as being intimately bound up with relationships (Dallos & Draper, 2010). Any particular 'problem' is not seen as a problem *per se*, but part of a larger process involving many other people, behaviours, and meanings (Campbell, Coldicott, & Kinsella, 1994). This contrasts with many psychotherapeutic approaches which focus primarily on the individual's intrapsychic experience. That said, intrapersonal experience is not denied: Minuchin (1974) suggested that the structural family therapist could be compared to a technician with a zoom lens, who could zoom in to study the individual's intrapsychic experience but could also observe with a broader focus on the system.

Several fundamental cybernetic ideas have endured throughout the history of systemic family therapy. There is an interest in how different members of a family *communicate* with each other: what and how things are expressed, and what goes unexpressed. Communication is the principal means by which different members of a system relate to each other and therefore a key area for intervention. Systemic family therapists are also reliably interested in the *(in)stability* of systems. 'Stuckness' or change are as likely to be the product of the flow of communication or information between parts of a system as of the intrinsic properties of any one person or part (Selvini Palazzoli et al., 1980). Finally, because specific behaviours and experiences are viewed as the collective achievement of many parts of a system, causation is considered to be *circular* rather than linear. This means that a cause cannot be traced backwards in a linear or reductionist fashion to an original source, meaning that any solutions to an apparent problem do not need to tackle the problem 'at source', but can be found in many places in a system; successful change is therefore achieved through the spiralling effects of feedback throughout the system (Penn, 1982). Families and therapists often seek the satisfaction and certainty of a linear explanation for problems, but this carries the risk of closing down opportunities for change that lie in unexpected places (Cecchin, 1987).

8.1.2 The stance of the therapist

A key feature of family therapy, especially in the function and purpose of formulation, is the emphasis on the therapist's use of 'self', and awareness of the stances they might take within sessions. It should be noted that there is little persuasive evidence for the relationship between this and the outcome of therapy (Horne, 1999), but it is generally accepted that the therapist should adopt a 'not-knowing' position and avoid imposing 'expert' therapeutic values (Amundson, Stewart, & Valentine, 1993).

This "not knowing" stance is usually considered necessary but not sufficient: the therapist may change stance depending on whether they wish to 'elicit' ideas and theories about the problem; 'probe' and offer new ideas or descriptions; 'contextualise' to make connections between a behaviour or idea and overall patterns in the system; 'match' to reflect back and empathise; or 'amplify' a particular idea, affect, theme, or behavioural sequence (Real, 1990). These stances are not exhaustive, but offer an illustration of how the therapist may shift their intentions and actions. The therapist should also be sensitive to their own experience as a potential tool that can further the therapeutic process (Rober, 2011). This has important implications for formulation: the therapist is not the fount of expert knowledge in which the solution will be found. Instead, they are a catalyst for change, using hypotheses to initiate and encourage change within a system.

8.1.3 Formulation Within Family Therapy

'Formulation' is not a term used in early family therapy literature, but has become more commonplace, perhaps particularly where clinical psychologists are also family therapists (e.g., Dallos & Draper, 2010). However, the processes of 'formulation' can be seen throughout the literature, as therapists drew connections between assessment information and systems theory to develop an understanding of problems and to devise an appropriate intervention. A seminal paper (Selvini Palazzoli et al., 1980) introduced three guidelines for family therapists, including 'hypothesising', which translates to what might be considered formulation. The Milan school were not concerned principally with the truth value of a hypothesis; rather, they were interested in a hypothesis' capacity to stimulate change in a system – it should offer the starting point for further investigation and should help the therapist to construct circular questions.

One legacy of the Milan approach is the caution provided to family therapists against 'marrying' our own hypotheses, at which point they cease to be helpful (Cecchin, 1987). Instead, they should revise their hypotheses in light of feedback from the family, and there is some evidence that therapists' reformulation of events and behaviours are an important component of therapy, in that they open up new possibilities for action and experiences (Sundet, 2011). The family therapist should never reach their final destination of complete understanding of their clients, as the not-yet-said is infinite (Rober, 1999).

Unlike some other approaches, family therapy does not have a range of pre-determined, problem-specific formulation models, although each of the schools offers specific ideas for formulating and intervening. There are no clear and detailed guidelines for family therapists to follow (Dallos & Draper, 2010), but rather a number of 'reference points' that might guide hypotheses (Boscolo & Bertrando, 1996). These are grounded in relevant theory, including ideas about attachment, power, and gender. Ideas about transitions in family boundaries (e.g., Wood & Talmon, 1983) and attachments (e.g., Byng-Hall, 2008) also offer frameworks for thinking about why difficulties arise within families.

8.1.4 Theories About 'Problems'

While all systemic approaches share the quite abstract principles described above, they vary significantly in the more concrete or mid-level concepts that they use to hypothesise why problems emerge within systems and how change might happen. These include behavioural patterns, belief systems, or emotional patterns within the family system, and the relationship between the family and wider cultural and political contexts (Vetere & Dallos, 2003). Systemic family therapists therefore draw upon a rich and diverse range of ideas, change might take place at a number of inter-related levels, and the formulation may well depend on the level of change that the therapist and family are working to create.

8.1.5 Structural Concepts

Structural perspectives focus on the organisation of family, including hierarchies and subsystems within the family, boundaries, rules, members' roles, and transactional patterns (Vetere, 2001). Family 'function' or 'dysfunction' would be determined according to how well or otherwise the family structure serves the developmental needs of the family members, and 'symptomatic behaviour' would be viewed as relating to some form of dysfunctional organisation (Colapinto, 1988). However, it is also assumed that the family has the competence to draw on inter- and intra-personal resources to bring about change, supported by the therapist (Vetere, 2001). The aim of therapy from a structural perspective is therefore to change the organisation of boundaries and related closeness or distance between family members and subsystems, in order to change each individual member's experience (Minuchin, 1974). The therapist aims to achieve this by supporting what is going well in the family, and joining family members to create changes in structures that are sustainable by challenging symptomatic behaviour, family structure, and/or family belief systems (Vetere, 2001).

8.1.6 Strategic Concepts

Strategic family therapy is so called because the therapist designs strategies in order to create change (Rosen, 2003). Within this approach, people are seen as inherently 'strategic' in attempting to influence each other, and problems are viewed as being embedded in repetitive interactional patterns (Dallos & Draper, 2010). Problems may be formulated as having a function within the system, such as maintaining system stability, and within therapy the therapist may 'reframe' the problem in terms of considering what function a particular problem might serve for members of the family.

An enduring strategic idea is that families may attempt to solve problems, but that repeatedly used ineffective solutions maintain problems, or give rise to new problems. When families present for help, it is often the ineffective solution, rather than the original problem, that is causing most difficulty. The aim of strategic approaches is to create behavioural change by disrupting unhelpful interactional patterns that inadvertently function to maintain the problem. The therapist contributes to the change process by encouraging experimentation to creatively solve challenges in novel ways, as well as encouraging what might be usually discouraged within the family, and emphasising and encouraging the clients' competence (Keim, 2012). The therapist might use a broad range of strategies and techniques designed to influence the specific family system. A range of example interventions are offered by Smith, Ruzgyte, and Spinks (2011).

8.1.7 Social Constructionist Concepts

The influence of social constructionism gave rise to even greater emphasis within family therapy on the role of language and multiple layers of context in creating and maintaining psychological distress. This emphasis owes a particular debt to the social constructionist argument that language, to a significant degree, constrains what can be thought and communicated about difficulties, and acts to help constitute subjective experience. Change within therapy was therefore seen to be brought about by the evolution of new meaning through dialogue (Anderson & Goolishian, 1988). The 'story' metaphor has had particular influence. This suggests that the 'problem saturated' stories that families frequently carry about their difficulties, whilst appearing to be convincing explanations, also serve to obscure possibilities for change. Therapists are concerned with assisting families to author alternative accounts of their lives that open up possibilities for change in action and experience.

8.2 Moving Towards Integration of Systemic Approaches to Formulation

In our formulation we draw upon an integrated model of systemic formulation first proposed by Vetere and Dallos (2003) and since discussed by Dallos and Draper (2010), and Dallos and Stedmon (2014). It proposes that assessment and formulation are two, interconnected processes referred to as 'analysis' and 'synthesis'. Analysis refers to the exploration of the nature of the family and their problems, while synthesis refers to 'starting to integrate the strands of information in preliminary hypotheses or formulations of the problem' (Vetere & Dallos, 2003, p. 75). The model attempts to reflect the differing emphasis placed by different phases of family therapy on patterns and processes, cognitions, language, and cultural contexts, and draw these together into one model, with five parts:

1. The problem – deconstruction
2. Problem-maintaining patterns and feedback loops
3. Beliefs and explanations
4. Emotions and attachments
5. Contextual factors

Our experience of using this model within clinical practice has highlighted its strengths but also potential challenges. Its breadth can be advantageous, in allowing consideration of a range of relevant factors drawn from the different schools of systemic family therapy. However, the model also throws open a challenge to the clinician in terms of where and how to focus within any of the five areas. There is no suggestion that the five parts of the model are intended to be considered sequentially, and in practice, there is often significant overlap between the five areas.

8.3 Empirical Evidence of Effectiveness

Family therapy has traditionally had an uncomfortable relationship with the decontextualized empiricism that characterizes much psychotherapy outcomes research. Arguably, research into therapies that focus on one individual offers clearer measurable outcomes than therapy with a relational focus. Not only might therapists and service commissioners have different views on outcomes, but different members of the same family may also have disparate views on what constitutes both the problem and the desired outcomes (Chenail *et al.*, 2011, cited Chenail, 2013). There are also challenges regarding what constitutes a measurable outcome, and how to capture therapeutic change that takes place during and outside therapy sessions, and both within and between individuals (Heatherington, Friedlander, & Greenberg, 2005).

Nevertheless, as the political climate of service provision has changed, there has been exponential growth in research during the past three decades (Sprenkle, 2012) and increasing interest in practitioners conducting research (e.g., Williams, Patterson, & Edwards, 2014). There is now evidence that family therapy can be effective for a wide range of difficulties across the life span (Stratton, 2005), although there remain significant gaps in empirical evidence for widely used approaches, including narrative therapy (Heatherington et al., 2005). Qualitative evidence has also begun emerging regarding families' experiences of therapy (e.g., Chenail et al., 2012). The evidence for one particular type of family therapy over another remains equivocal. Why family therapy works, or when and under what circumstances, remains "shrouded in mystery", and there is little to refute the hypothesis that family therapy works because of common mechanisms of change across all approaches (Sprenkle, 2012, p. 25). These common factors include conceptualising difficulties in relational terms, working to disrupt dysfunctional relational patterns, expanding the direct treatment system, and expanding the therapeutic alliance (Sprenkle, Davis, & Lebow, 2009), and support an argument for the integrated approach outlined above. It is also important that research evidence in isolation does not determine clinical decisions made by therapists, who should integrate the evidence-base with the culture, values, and preferences of clients, and their own clinical expertise, in order to deliver competent therapy (Chenail, 2013).

8.4 Critique

In a certain sense, systemic family therapy has been its own strongest critic. One reason for the fractured evolution of this approach is the willingness of practitioners to criticise their particular school, and draw upon a range of ideas to inform these criticisms. Implicit assumptions about 'normal families' underpinning earlier structural approaches, ethical concerns that a therapist might seek to be 'neutral' when particular family members may be oppressing or abusing other family members, and other aspects of family therapy have been critically and rightfully scrutinised (Dallos & Draper, 2010). However, many of the attributes of systemic family therapy described above might be considered potentially problematic, either as a basis for formulation, or more widely as a school of psychotherapy demanding a significant place within psychological healthcare. The emphasis upon the inter-personal certainly appears to have resulted in an under-theorisation of intra-psychic phenomena, and the lack of models to explain the aetiology and development of specific problems, whilst consistent with a systemic epistemology, means family therapists must work from broad principles rather than a precise 'recipe'. This perhaps compares unfavourably with the testability and consistency offered by increasingly prescriptive cognitive-behavioural approaches to formulation and therapy, and potentially carries the risk that family therapy constructs and interventions can be used by some clinicians in an ineffective or theoretically contradictory manner.

Clinical work with multiple persons and teams of therapists may also be alien to clients expecting an individual approach, and the use of teams of therapists might be considered costly by service commissioners. However, research examining the costs of such approaches at the two-year follow-up stage suggests that family therapy is no more costly, and may be substantially less costly, than other therapies (Stratton, 2011).

8.5 Formulation in Action

Below, we illustrate the process of formulation in three stages. First we consider our initial responses to the case. Second, we describe an 'analysis' of some potential systemic hypotheses following the five areas described above. Finally, we present a distilled 'synthesis' of these ideas.

In keeping with the use of self and reflexivity in family therapy, we gave thought to the information that appeared most salient to each of us individually, considered our initial positions in relation to different members of the family, and how these might create 'blind spots' or potential biases during formulation and therapy. Anna's initial thoughts were as follows:

I was struck by the apparent lack of affirmation Molly received from her parents, in contrast to my own experiences as a daughter. Molly's wish to make her parents proud because of their emphasis on success was in common with my own wish to make my parents proud through achievement. However, I was fortunate to draw on emotional and practical resources from my parents. Initially, I found it difficult not to align myself with Molly 'against' her parents for expecting her to succeed, but seeming to 'fail' to provide the foundations from which she could achieve. I would need to remain cognisant of this within sessions in order not to privilege her perspective over that of her parents. I also have strong feelings against the medicalisation of distress; I was conscious that I felt angry that it seemed the systems around Molly may be more willing to frame her as 'histrionic' or 'ill', rather than consider how sexual abuse or familial and social circumstances may have contributed to her distress.

Mike's initial thoughts were as follows:

> I was curious about when (if ever) relationship difficulties had not been such a significant part of Molly's life. On first reading the case summary, a 'problem saturated' story of Molly's life seems unavoidable. Her descriptions of relationship difficulties and disappointments at various stages of her life make this appear to be a long-standing and continuous problem. Her experience of being sexually abused and the lack of a supportive response to this might well account for some of these difficulties. However, this story might risk neglecting important contextual aspects of each significant relationship experience, although I'm aware that this response might constitute 'wishful thinking' on my part, and inquiring after 'exceptions' to troubling experiences must never be allowed to be construed as a lack of appreciation of the seriousness of a person's dif-

ficulties. I was also concerned with Molly's apparent reluctance to discuss her experience of sexual abuse. There might be any number of potential hypotheses to explain this reluctance, but I would be interested in how we might talk about 'talking about the abuse', in order that any discussion of such a potentially significant experience does not compound the apparent harm of the lack of response to the abuse when it occurred.

To best illustrate the process of formulation in systemic practice, we begin by sharing our development of many potential systemic hypotheses. The information most pertinent to the formulation is that which gives insight into the relationships between Molly and her family/social systems, both past and present. In many respects, information about presenting 'problems', such as eating and sleeping patterns, would be less pertinent to us, as these would be seen as a manifestation of relational difficulties. However, they must not be dismissed, as they may be viewed as 'the problem' by Molly and connect to her goal to 'get better'. Changes in these reported difficulties may also provide an opportunity to measure change.

8.5.1 Deconstruction of the Problem

We agreed to prioritise the deconstruction of the problem. This would include consideration of how different members of the family define the problem, how the problem affects relationships and vice versa, for whom the problem is most difficult, the life history of the problem, and exceptions to the problem (Vetere & Dallos, 2003). At this point, we only have information from Molly, which would be a significant limitation. We would want to seek information from family members by inviting them to a family session.

On the whole, Molly frames the problem and the onus for change as located within her, e.g., referring to needing help to "sort (herself) out". There are many indications of her perceived personal failings, such as being unattractive, underachieving, unable to fit in, and unable to meet the sexual needs of potential partners. Even where problems have arisen in the context of other people behaving in particular ways towards her, Molly frequently frames the problem as her reaction to them. Similarly, family members appear to locate the problem within Molly, viewing her as "overly emotional". To us, the interpersonal nature of Molly's difficulties seems evident throughout her history and current concerns, and our first hypothesis is that the array of difficulties Molly describes over time are signs of a struggle to 'fit in' with her family and wider social system. Moving towards a more systemic deconstruction of the problem may be a challenge, as we would be starting at a very different position to Molly and members of her system. This also highlights some of the inherent tensions within contemporary family therapy, as our fundamental hypothesis that the problem is relational may be seen to contradict the adoption of a 'not knowing position'. As family therapy values and allows for multiple perspectives to be heard, we would not seek to dismiss individualised conceptualisations of Molly's difficulties, but to open up the possibility that Molly's difficulties may be *both* located in her (through their construction within the language of the system) *and* relational in their origin and maintenance.

There do appear to be some exceptions to Molly's difficulties, including: success at school; forming relationships (both with men and colleagues); gaining employment; initially enjoying living independently in her flat and being motivated; and some positive relationships with staff during her inpatient stay. Further, some of the problematic processes identified below might very well be intended to solve other problems. Any such exceptions or good intentions might be drawn upon in both the development of hypotheses and during interventions, but remain undeveloped and relatively untouched at the stage of assessment.

8.5.2 Problem-maintaining Patterns and Feedback Loops

Here, we would be interested in considering the structures of the family and any repetitive behavioural patterns based on feedback loops within the system (Vetere & Dallos, 2003). Drawing on structural family theory, it could be suggested that the boundaries between family members seem to be rigid to the point of disconnection (Minuchin, 1974), and have led to a perceived lack of emotional connectedness between family members. However, in light of Anna's aforementioned reflections, it would be important to understand the boundaries of the family from the perspective of each of its members, rather than imposing the therapist's own, potentially biased, perspective.

We would not argue that the kind of family structure described by Molly is always problematic, but that in some circumstances there is a poor fit. In Molly's case, this structure might have significantly reduced the family's ability to respond to her experience of sexual abuse in a constructive fashion. Indeed, Molly herself reported feeling constrained from disclosing the abuse, and her family appear not to have been alert to any changes in emotion or behaviour that Molly most likely experienced after the abuse.

The family organisation may have compounded these difficulties later. The transition out of the family home to university was difficult for Molly. Transitions such as a child leaving home are often stressful for the system, and the family will sometimes respond by clinging to old roles and patterns (Wood & Talmon, 1983). In addition, there is evidence that parent-daughter boundaries are connected to young adult females' development of an independent identity (Fullinwider-Bush & Jacobvitz, 1993). Molly attempted to follow a 'normative' path of going to university, but "failed" to take this step towards autonomy, relative to both the family norms and expectations (achieved by her sister), and broader social norms. It may be that this context perpetuated the organisational family pattern of Molly being identified as "overly emotional" by other family members.

The primary feedback loop we would be interested in focusing on relates to Molly's expression of emotion and need for closeness, and the apparent consequential rejection by others, which may lead to an escalation in both distress and rejection. An alternative is for Molly to suppress the expression of her emotional needs, but this may lead to other manifestations of distress. We also considered a feedback loop in which Molly aims to please others but has never quite succeeded or 'failed enough'; her successes have not been sufficient to achieve the kind of recognition she seeks from her parents (in particular), but neither has she failed sufficiently to prompt experimentation with other goals or life plans.

Two other possible feedback loops were identified that might be of relevance, but which will not be the key focus of the present formulation. The first related to Molly's difficulties having sexual relationships, leading her to avoid intimacy. This in turn may lead others to view her as not seeking intimacy, thus maintaining the difficulty by reducing opportunities to develop sexual relationships. The second related to Molly withholding information about being sexually abused from her family through fear of 'wrecking the family'. The family is therefore denied the possibility to respond in any way, maintaining Molly's fear and anticipation of a catastrophic response, and potentially facilitating further withholding of information.

8.5.3 Beliefs and Explanations

We would also explore different levels of beliefs about the problem and what should be done about it, including family members' perceptions, and socio-cultural beliefs and discourses from outside of the family (Vetere & Dallos, 2003). There appears to be congruence between Molly's belief that she is not coping, and the family belief that she is 'over emotional'. These beliefs might also link with discourses in mental health services about individuals who may be discussed as having a 'personality disorder'. The interaction between these beliefs at different levels may contribute to a dominant story that the problem is located within Molly, and is related to her personal failings, rather than having a relational aetiology. It is striking that these explanations do not draw upon Molly's experience of sexual abuse and the lack of a protective response to this. Further, these explanations do not really account for exceptions when Molly has been able to function well and relate to others.

8.5.4 Emotions and Attachments

In deconstructing the problem, we were particularly drawn to the hypothesis that expressions of emotion were discouraged within the family and that Molly's emotional expression led her to be viewed as "overly emotional". This is a pattern that appears to have occurred in Molly's other relationships, and in the initial response she received from mental health services. Molly's expression of emotion might be helpfully understood as an attachment behaviour with an *intended* function of securing relational safety and closeness, but an *actual* effect of troubling her relationships and triggering further distress.

8.5.5 Contextual Factors

These factors relate to resources, the history of the problem, environmental factors, extended family, role of professional agencies, and cultural discourses (Vetere & Dallos, 2003). These have largely been addressed in the previous sections of the model so will not be considered further here.

8.5.6 Initial Formulation

The analysis above using the integrated framework helped us to consider a range of systemic ideas and theories that may be relevant to developing a formulation of Molly and her difficulties. However, it already appears "like an overwhelming kaleidoscope of factors" that need to be synthesised into a manageable formulation (Vetere & Dallos, 2003, p. 81). In reality, we would not be sharing hypotheses with the family based only on information from one family member. Instead, we would work from a position of curiosity with the family to develop and revise hypotheses that may be useful in introducing potential for change. Hypotheses would be shared with the family soon after they came to mind, to lead to the family discussing the idea (Byng-Hall, 2008) and to facilitate opportunities to respond to their feedback in line with the principle of circularity (Selvini Palazzoli et al., 1980).

Molly's identity is dominated by beliefs or a dominant 'story' that she falls short of her own and other people's standards and expectations, both in terms of relationships and achievements. These beliefs seem to have developed through early experiences of family relationships and continue to affect her relationships with others within and outside of the family. Molly is more open about expressing her emotional needs than her parents. Molly's mother in particularly seems to focus on achievements rather than emotions in her interactions with Molly, perhaps because she was keen for her daughter to be 'successful'. The problem maintaining feedback loop below outlines the relationship between Molly's emotional expression and her family's view of her:

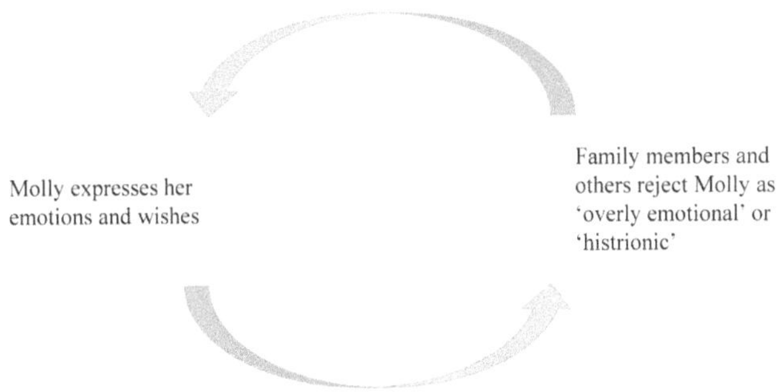

The problem may escalate as Molly experiences increased distress in response to rejection, or expresses her emotional needs in other ways (including some of the behaviours she sees as problematic), which may in turn lead to further actual or anticipated rejection. Molly's experience of sexual abuse, and her fear of rejection if this is disclosed, may also contribute to this problem-maintaining feedback loop.

However, it is important to note that the formulation remains tentative and could change significantly when different perspectives from other family members are put forward.

8.5.7 Intervention Objectives

The objective of the therapy would be to achieve positive change for Molly in the areas that she has identified. However, in keeping with the wide range of options available for change within systemic practice, the 'specific' mechanisms of change are potentially still broad – creating change in any of the behavioural patterns, belief systems, or emotional patterns within the family system and in the relationship between the family and wider cultural and political contexts (Vetere & Dallos, 2003). Given the complexity of even small social systems, how change unfolds must be regarded as uncertain. Rather than prescribing precise targets for change, formulation in systemic practice suggests areas for therapists to focus upon. Skilfully done, these therapeutic efforts will incite changes in patterns of communication, belief, and behaviour in the areas of most concern to the family.

Ultimately, Molly and her family must determine whether the objective of achieving positive change has been met. In systemic practice families are frequently invited to comment on whether any progress is being made. 'Scaling questions' are a well-known technique of monitoring progress towards problem resolution, using a ten-point scale (Berg & de Shazer, 1993). To aid the measurement of change, we could also use a well-established contemporary measure of family functioning and change, such as the SCORE-15 – derived from the original SCORE-40 (Stratton, Bland, Janes, & Lask, 2010, see aft.org.uk/view/score.html).

8.5.8 Intervention Plan

In keeping with a systemic approach, here we identify our starting point for therapy and likely approach to the work. Anything more specific would assume that our ideas and practice would not change across the therapy, which is certainly not the case.

A systemic intervention would most likely face two initial challenges: firstly, joining with the family to promote a family level solution to something that is perceived to be an individual's problem; and secondly, beginning the work with a systemic hypothesis that challenges key family beliefs. Our starting point would be to invite the whole family into a therapy session, if they were willing, in order to focus on the relational aspects of Molly's difficulties. As therapists, we would aim to create a secure therapeutic base for the family; the initial session may last an hour and a half or more, to "allow time for difficult issues to emerge with some intensity and have some chance of being addressed" (Byng-Hall, 2008, p. 138). Molly would also need to be given individual time, apart from her family, to consider how and when her experience of abuse may, or may not, be discussed.

A range of question types would be used within sessions to facilitate 'interventive interviewing' (Tomm, 1988) – a style of asking therapeutic questions that potentially fosters change in a system. Lineal questions would be used first in order to establish the definition of the problems from the perspective of each family member. Circular questions would then be used more frequently to compel the family to experience the circularity of their family system, to shift away from more linear stances, leading to increased perceived membership of the problem (Penn, 1982). This would open up the possibility for new stories to develop within the family system based on familial patterns rather than "truths" and facts (Cecchin, 1987). We would also be interested in identifying patterns or scripts within the family that highlight how family roles have developed (Byng-Hall, 2008), and may use genograms of wider family relationships to reveal broader patterns (McGoldrick, Gerson, & Petry, 2008).

If within-session exploration supported the initial formulation outlined above, the aim of therapy would be to disrupt these patterns by focusing on both how Molly expresses her emotional needs, and how others respond to her. In addition to the above, we might make use of strategic questions, which are designed to influence the client or family in a specific way, in this case by reducing the likelihood of them continuing along the same problematic path (Tomm, 1988). Reflexive questions would also be used to encourage the family to generate their own connections and solutions in their own manner and time (Tomm, 1988). By generating alternative ways of behaving, and fostering alternative beliefs about the behaviour within the family system, we would be optimistic that beneficial therapeutic change would be forthcoming. However, if change within the system was difficult to enact, we would revisit our hypotheses and formulation in order to identify any crucial information we may have missed, and reflect on any assumptions that were made that may have been erroneous or that led to a less effective way of working with this particular family system.

Thomas Schröder, Angela Cooper & Rohan Naidoo

8.6 Systemic Family Therapy Formulation: Critical Commentary

"The map is not the territory" warned Alfred Korzybski more than 80 years ago, and the metaphor of the map helps to portray some of the issues involved in critically reviewing a case formulation developed from a theoretical framework different to one's own. Just as a topographical and a geological map will show different features of the same terrain, so the different observational perspectives entailed by the various therapeutic orientations afford different representations of the same clinical phenomena. Some discrepancies are simply a matter of nomenclature, allowing for straight translations between alternative formulations; others represent different emphases in observation. We can compare divergent maps and even enter into their particular viewpoints if they share sufficient common characteristics. By contrast, we would have difficulties recognising a territory represented by aboriginal songlines, and our pets presumably have precise olfactory maps of our homes to which we have as little access as they have to our carefully drawn floor plans. What allows us as psychologists to mediate between our varying therapeutic perspectives are common clinical observations, which – although constrained by our interpretative scaffolds – are relatively constant, and our shared commitment to paying attention to evidence, both from the narrower clinical and the broader psychology sources, even though we may argue about what should count as legitimate evidence.

Regarding this latter point, we think that the authors of this chapter could have been bolder in arguing not only for the possibility, but indeed for the necessity of using multiple sources of evidence. While systemic approaches and ISTDP share misgivings about the 'decontextualized relationship that characterises much psychotherapy outcome research', there are serviceable alternatives. Contemporary ISTDP researchers make extensive use of single case study designs for investigating both outcome and process. With this in mind, there is no good reason why the processes and contexts characterising successful systemic family therapy should remain "shrouded in mystery". An allegiance to maintaining openness to multiple explanations and scepticism towards assertions of 'the truth' should not lead us to give up on the search for truths, partial though they may be.

Using the therapist's own experience as a potential source of information is an idea that appears to be shared by psychodynamic and systemic practitioners, be that in order to 'further the therapeutic process' as suggested in this chapter, or to gain better understanding, both cognitively and emotionally. To record the authors' differential initial reactions to the clinical material is a promising start, but we wonder whether it has been made the most of here. There is a clear contrast between Anna's emotional – and in part visceral – reaction to the material, based on her personal history and early experience as well as on her current values, and Mike's more cognitive response, driven by intellectual curiosity but tempered by caveats about potential biases. It may be that these are gendered reactions or that they are simply representative of two of the repertoires at the therapist's disposal – feeling and thinking. It is plausible, however, that they might pick up a tension within Molly, between her emotional needs and her wish to please by intellectual achievement, as later alluded to in the description of the 'primary feedback loop'. Such an intrapsychic experience would of course be played out in, and reciprocally strengthened by, its interpersonal parallels. To explore this possibility further, we wish that the authors had drawn on the two other repertoires available to them – acting and relating. It would have been good to have had access to the dialogue between them, exploring their different reactions rather than filing them away as potential sources of trouble. Having two (or more) people interacting in responding to the same material is a valuable resource between co-therapists or in a reflective team; it might have equally helped to deepen the reader's access to the systemic formulations. This could have also led us into a discussion of intersubjectivity (to what extent the drawing of the map *creates* the territory), which should be a particular strength of the systemic approach and an area that other viewpoints could learn from. Though an area of debate among psychodynamic therapists, it is not usually addressed within the literature on ISTDP.

Most notably, we were struck by the relative neglect of specific emotions in the formulations. It is not clear whether in systemic approaches emotions would be seen purely as epiphenomena, as in behavioural theory, or regarded as central, as they would be in process-experiential and psychodynamic approaches. 'Emotions and attachments' had been listed as one of the five areas that an integrated model of systemic formulation would need to pay attention to, but it appears that they are not an important component in this chapter, maybe mirroring Molly's family and their attitudes towards emotional expressiveness. 'Distress' is a rather imprecise description for a reaction that may encompass anger, sadness, disgust, shame, guilt, humiliation, and fear, among others. One might argue that such feelings are intrapsychic experiences and therefore outside the purview of an interactional perspective; however, such a position would overlook the concept of emotions being reciprocally determined, either in a symmetrical or complementary fashion, as first postulated by interpersonal theorists.

Finally, we would want to acknowledge the broad areas of overlap between our outlook and the systemic perspective. Critical reviews invite the 'narcissism of small differences' that often characterises the exchanges between the different therapeutic tribes. Research evidence tells us that theoretical orientation has a negligible influence on outcome variance, but as clinicians we need the containment that a coherent perspective affords us when faced with the uncertainties and challenges of our daily practice. We hope the dialogue in this chapter and this book helps all of us to broaden our repertoires – emotional, relational, cognitive, and behavioural – when we engage in psychological therapies.

Anna Tickle & Michael Rennoldson

8.7 Author Response

We would like to signal our agreement with the key sentiment of the critique; that we have far more in common than apart.

When focussing upon our differences, the ISTDP authors have identified in our formulation an absence that is arguably seen across much, though not all, systemic thought and practice – namely a lack of a precise classification of emotion. One potential response that we might adopt as systemic practitioners is to make greater efforts to incorporate interpersonal theories of emotion, such as attachment theory or ideas from the psychodynamic tradition. However, we are drawn to a different response that reflects another point of difference identified in the critique. Many contemporary systemic practitioners do believe that the map 'creates' the territory. That is to say, the ideas and words we use to name and interpret experience become constitutive of that experience. From this flows a reluctance to name or specify emotion at the level of detail promoted within ISTDP at the stage of formulation. Rather, we might invite Molly and other family members to 'name' these experiences for themselves. Differences identified between family members in conceptualising emotional experiences would be seen not as problematic, but as a potential resource for therapeutic change. At this stage in the formulation, the feedback loop that offers a general interactional pattern relating to emotional expression could be a starting point from which to identify situations or examples in which specific emotions could be named and discussed.

The critique also encouraged greater use of research to investigate both outcome and process. There is undoubtedly a need for systemic practice to develop a much more substantial body of process and outcome research. However, finding a form of credible and purposeful research that remains consistent with an interest in multiple perspectives and a model of circular causation is a challenge.

We also agree that it would have been useful for us to present some of the dialogue between us about our initial responses to the material, although our rationale for this would be different to that suggested. The critique saw it as plausible that our two different reactions – one more 'emotional', the other more 'cognitive' – might represent a tension within Molly. From our perspective, the different reactions would not be seen to reflect the internal state(s) of the client, but instead to reflect the 'use of self' encouraged within systemic therapy. Observing intersubjectivity in action could have given insight into how multiple perspectives might shape a systemic formulation, including potential benefits of different therapists' world views compensating for each other's 'blind spots'. Equally, it could raise some questions about the interactional patterns and issues between team members, such as whether some are seen to hold more power and influence than others and potential reasons for this.

References

Amundson, J., Stewart, K., & Valentine, L. (1993). Temptations of power and certainty. *Journal of Marital and Family Therapy, 19*(2), 111-123.

Anderson, H., & Goolishian, H. A. (1988). Human systems as linguistic systems: Preliminary and evolving ideas about the implications for clinical theory. *Family Process, 27*(4), 371-393.

Berg, I. K., & de Shazer, S. (1993). Making numbers talk: Language in therapy. In S. Friedman (Ed.), *The new language of change: Constructive collaboration in psychotherapy*, (pp. 5-24). New York: Guilford Press.

Boscolo, L., & Bertrando, P. (1996). *Systemic therapy with individuals*. London: Karnac Books.

Byng-Hall, J. (2008). The crucial roles of attachment in family therapy. *Journal of Family Therapy, 30*(2), 129-146.

Campbell, D., Coldicott, T., & Kinsella, K. (1994). *Systemic work with organizations: A new model for managers and change agents*. London: Karnac Books.

Cecchin, G. (1987). Hypothesizing, circularity, and neutrality revisited: An invitation to curiosity. *Family Process, 26*(4), 405-413.

Chenail, R. J. (2013). Evidence and efficacy issues. In A. Rambo, C. West, A. Schooley & T. V. Boyd (Eds.), *Family therapy review: Contrasting contemporary models* (pp. 25-32). London: Routledge.

Chenail, R. J., George, S. S., Wulff, D., Duffy, M., Scott, K. W., & Tomm, K. (2012). Clients' relational conceptions of conjoint couple and family therapy quality: A grounded formal theory. *Journal of Marital and Family Therapy, 38*(1), 241-264.

Colapinto, J. (1988). Teaching the structural way. In H. A. Liddle, D. C. Breunlin & R. C. Schwartz (Eds.), *Handbook of family therapy training and supervision* (pp. 17-37). New York: The Guildford Press.

Dallos, R., & Draper, R. (2010). *An introduction to family therapy: Systemic theory and practice*. McGraw-Hill International.

Dallos, R., & Stedmon, J. (2014). Systemic formulation: mapping the family dance. In L. Johnstone & R. Dallos (Eds.), *Formulation in psychology and psychotherapy: Making sense of people's problems* (pp. 67-95). London: Routledge.

Falloon, I. R. H. (1988). *Behavioural Family Therapy: A Workbook*. London: Routledge.

Fullinwider-Bush, N., & Jacobvitz, D. B. (1993). The transition to young adulthood: Generational boundary dissolution and female identity development. *Family Process, 32*(1), 87-103.

Heatherington, L., Friedlander, M. L., & Greenberg, L. (2005). Change process research in couple and family therapy: methodological challenges and opportunities. *Journal of Family Psychology, 19*(1), 18-27.

Horne, K. B. (1999). The relationship of the self of the therapist to therapy process and outcome: Are some questions better left unanswered? *Contemporary Family Therapy, 21*(3), 385-403.

Keim, J. (2012). Strategic family therapy. In A. Rambo, C. West, A. Schooley & T. V. Boyd (Eds.), *Family therapy review: Contrasting contemporary models* (pp. 89-93). London: Routledge.

McGoldrick, M., Gerson, R., & Petry, S. S. (2008). *Genograms: Assessment and intervention* (3rd ed.). New York: WW Norton & Company.

Minuchin, S. (1974). *Families and Family Therapy*. Harvard University Press.

Penn, P. (1982). Circular questioning. *Family Process, 21*(3), 267-280.

Real, T. (1990). The therapeutic use of self in constructionist/systemic therapy. *Family Process, 29*(3), 255-272.

Rober, P. (1999). The therapist's inner conversation in family therapy practice: Some ideas about the self of the therapist, therapeutic impasse, and the process of reflection. *Family Process, 38*(2), 209-228.

Rober, P. (2011). The therapist's experiencing in family therapy practice. *Journal of Family Therapy, 33*(3), 233-255.
Rosen, K. H. (2003). Strategic family therapy. In L. J. Hecker & J. L. Wetchler (Eds.), *An introduction to marriage and family therapy*. Abingdon, UK: Taylor & Francis.
Selvini Palazzoli, M., Boscolo, L., Cecchin, G., & Prata, G. (1980). Hypothesizing—circularity—neutrality: Three guidelines for the conductor of the session. *Family Process, 19*(1), 3-12.
Smith, T. N., Ruzgyte, E., & Spinks, D. (2011). Strategic Family Therapy. In L. Metcalf (Ed.), *Marriage and Family Therapy: A Practice-Oriented Approach* (pp. 255-286). New York: Springer Publishing Company.
Sprenkle, D. H. (2012). Intervention research in couple and family therapy: A methodological and substantive review and an introduction to the special issue. *Journal of Marital and Family Therapy, 38*(1), 3-29.
Sprenkle, D. H., Davis, S. D., & Lebow, J. L. (2009). *Common factors in couple and family therapy: The overlooked foundation for effective practice*. London: Guilford Press.
Stratton, P. (2005). *Report on the evidence base of systemic family therapy*. UK: Association for Family Therapy.
Stratton, P. (2011). *The evidence base of systemic family and couples therapies*. UK: Association for Family Therapy.
Stratton, P., Bland, J., Janes, E., & Lask, J. (2010). Developing an indicator of family function and a practicable outcome measure for systemic family and couple therapy: The SCORE. *Journal of Family Therapy, 32*(3), 232-258.
Sundet, R. (2011). Collaboration: Family and therapist perspectives of helpful therapy. *Journal of Marital and Family Therapy, 37*(2), 236-249.
Tomm, K. (1988). Interventive interviewing: Part III. Intending to ask lineal, circular, strategic, or reflexive questions? *Family Process, 27*(1), 1-15.
Vetere, A. (2001). Structural family therapy. *Child Psychology and Psychiatry Review, 6*(03), 133-139.
Vetere, A., & Dallos, R. (2003). *Working Systemically with Families: Formulation, Intervention and Evaluation*. London: Karnac.
Von Bertalanffy, L. (1950). An outline of general system theory. *British Journal for the Philosophy of Science, 1*, 139-164.
Watzlawick, P., Weakland, J. H., & Fisch, R. (1974). *Change; Principles of Problem Formation and Problem Resolution*. New York: W. W. Norton.
Williams, L., Patterson, J., & Edwards, T. M. (2014). *Clinician's Guide to Research Methods in Family Therapy: Foundations of Evidence-Based Practice*. London: Guilford Publications.
Wood, B., & Talmon, M. (1983). Family boundaries in transition: A search for alternatives. *Family Process, 22*(3), 347-357.

Rachel Sabin-Farrell & Roger Bretherton

9 Body-Centred Psychotherapy (BCP)

Body-Centred Psychotherapy (BCP) takes as its starting point the principle that all psychological experiences, pleasant and unpleasant, are embodied experiences (Keleman, 1981). As philosophers are keen to remind us, we do not just *have* bodies, we *are* bodies (Marcel, 1964). The world around us from conception onwards affects and leaves its mark upon the body; a point increasingly emphasised in developmental interpersonal neurobiology (Siegel, 2010) and developmental psychology (Gerhardt, 2006). For this reason, BCP asserts that the body deserves great attention in clinical practice.

Recognising the importance of the body is not unique to BCP however. Therapies from the cognitive-behavioural tradition, for example, stress awareness of physiological phenomena and include bodily awareness in their formulations (e.g., Padesky & Greenberger, 1995). Eye Movement Desensitisation and Reprocessing (EMDR) considers physical sensations a central part of the trauma treatment protocol (Shapiro, 2001). The humanistic school of psychotherapy equally pays great attention to the body. Gendlin, a philosopher working alongside Carl Rogers, developed 'focussing', a technique by which an embodied *felt-sense* expresses itself in language (Gendlin, 2003). Likewise, several of the therapeutic experiments designed by Frederick Perls aim to foster awareness of habitual gestures and bodily responses (Kepner, 1987). Similarly, psychodynamic approaches demonstrate interest in bodily experience, and the muscular tensions and somatic symptoms habitually reported by analytic patients (Reich, 1980; Young, 2006). Some psychodynamic practitioners have even been so bold as to state that the body *is* the unconscious (Lowen, 1975). Contemporary BCP draws upon, or incorporates, many approaches, but in recent decades it has undergone considerable theoretical development. Carroll (2003) suggests that there is a 'cultural and paradigm shift' towards recognising the embodiment of psychological processes and therefore the importance of the role of the body in therapy. Research on psychological trauma (e.g., van der Kolk, 1996, 2014) and the neuropsychological literature with links to attachment theory (Schore, 2003; Solomon & Siegel, 2003), has further driven BCP to gather a repertoire of therapeutic techniques, many of which are outlined below.

BCP is therefore most accurately viewed as a cluster of psychotherapies rather than a single approach (Totton, 2003) and can be usefully grouped into three discernible models: the *adjustment* model, which views the correct aligning of the body as a way to psychological health; the *trauma* model, which holds therapy to be a process of abreaction or emotional expression in which past trauma is released from being trapped in the body; and the *process* model, which aims to sensitively facilitate the healing or psychological growth process latent in the body. Each of these models has its advantages and drawbacks, but many contemporary systems of Body Psychotherapy are a synthesis of these approaches.

The term BCP in this chapter is therefore used to denote an approach which is a synthesis of these three models and is derived from, but not confined to, that elaborated by Ron Kurtz (1990), often called Hakomi (a Native American term paraphrased as 'to be well in all one's worlds'). We draw to some extent on the historical BCP literature of Character Analysis (Reich, 1980) and Bioenergetics (Lowen, 1975). We incorporate more recent contributions to the BCP literature from Character Styles (Johnson, 1994), Trauma Therapy (Levine, 1997; Rothschild, 2000), Attachment (Schore, 2003), Focussing (Campbell & McMahon, 1997; Friedman, 2007), and Executive Development (Cotter, 1996). We also anticipate further developments in the pioneering work of The Sensorimotor Psychotherapy Institute (www.sensorimotorpsychotherapy.org), only some of which have yet found their way into the public domain in the form of articles and book-length monographs. But in using the term Body-Centred Psychotherapy we are primarily drawing on the approach outlined by Kurtz, with some notable additions from the other models.

One of the unique theoretical contributions of the BCP approach is the notion of 'character strategy', a set of short-hand characterisations that aid the therapist to quickly understand the habitual ways in which their client relates to the world. Character strategies are not personality types but rather themes that can be identified in people. Any given client can present with several character strategies in operation. They do not represent a person's identity but rather habitual patterns of relating to the world. Over the last century, various schemes of character strategies have been proposed in BCP (Cotter, 1996; Johnson, 1994; Lowen, 1975; Reich, 1980). In the Hakomi approach, Ron Kurtz (1990) developed a roster of eight strategies, each named functionally rather than pathologically. He viewed character strategy as a "strength developed to the point of imbalance" which becomes "a weakness" on the basis that "every function overly developed in one direction leaves another direction undeveloped" (p. 40). Ogden added a sensitive/emotional character strategy to the eight put forward by Kurtz (Fisher & Boreham, 2014a). Understanding the character strategies, and how they influence the organisation of present moment experience, is a key part of the theory and practice of Hakomi and Sensorimotor Psychotherapy and will be utilised in the formulation below.

9.1 Empirical Evidence

In terms of evidence-base, BCP as a movement has tended to eschew randomised controlled trials (RCTs) and other clinical research methods. Dinas (2012) highlighted the difficulty of constructing useful outcome measures or psychometric instruments when therapeutic changes are difficult to put into words. In addition, it is challenging to devise an RCT with a therapy that tracks the client so closely and alters technique based on the in-session experience of the client and in-vivo experimentation. Similar problems of evaluation are reported in other therapeutic approaches that construct a bespoke treatment strategy for each client (Yalom, 2009).

Nevertheless, some single-case and anecdotal evidence for BCP effectiveness has been accrued. Individual clients report the benefits of the approach (Dinas, 2012; Fisher & Ogden, 2009), as do participants in a stabilization group intervention (Langmuir, Kirsh, & Classen, 2012). In addition to this, clinicians in the trauma field endorse the theoretical necessity of focusing on the body (Lanius, Lanius, Fisher, & Ogden, 2006; Levine, 1997; van der Kolk, 1996, 2014) and have published case examples (Rothschild, 2003). However, further studies on BCP are needed to establish the evidence-base for this approach.

9.2 Formulation in Action

The formulation presented in this chapter therefore uses the term 'body centred psychotherapy' (BCP) to refer to Hakomi and Sensorimotor Psychotherapies. Within this approach, key factors to inform an initial formulation include: indications of past trauma (either event-based trauma or attachment-related developmental trauma), character strategy, and how present moment experience is organised, and could provide a frame to access 'core material' for intervention.

Our initial hypotheses were that Molly's main issues were driven by character strategy developed in her early and subsequent attachments and relationships. However, there may also be traumatic roots to her difficulties.

9.2.1 Character Strategies

When looking for possible character strategies, we pay attention to how they currently appear and play out in relationships, work, decision making and other key areas of a person's life. In the assessment phase, we would assess particularly how the character strategies are manifested in the body and what the current 'felt sense' is within the session when attention is paid to elements of the story or difficulty being described. From the case description, we will highlight certain information which may indicate certain character strategies. However, accurate identification of character strategies requires a therapist to be in contact with a patient (Glazer & Friedman, 2009), and any conclusions drawn from a written account are therefore reflective of working hypotheses.

On first reading it appears that Molly exhibits what BCP would call Sensitive-Withdrawn (S/W) character strategy. She takes refuge in withdrawing from people as it feels threatening to be in contact with others. The other main character strategy evidenced in the case is named Expressive-Clinging (E/C) in the BCP nomenclature.

This is a strategy that attempts to maintain contact with others by dramatising to sustain attention. The indications of clinginess in relationships and words such as 'dramatic' used by her parents to describe Molly give a clue to this strategy. While other strategies may also be present or uncovered during therapy, the initial formulation stresses the tension exhibited in Molly between her dominant S/W presentation and the signals of an E/C strategy. While the S/W strategy seeks to withdraw from others, the E/C strategy clings to them. They therefore represent conflicting needs in Molly and it is possible that she is pulled between the opposite desires of seeking separation yet needing togetherness. This inner conflict is seen in contrasting behaviour, cognitions, emotions, body posture, inner sensation, movement, and five sense perception – what Kurtz (1990) terms the 'core organisers' of present moment experience.

9.2.2 Trauma

During the assessment and therapy process, signs of the remnants of unresolved past trauma would be tracked in the body. The sexual abuse disclosed is said to have occurred when Molly was aged nine, so traumatic elements would be considered in the context of developing character, also acknowledging the additional affects the trauma may have had on Molly, and how this is held in her body. It is difficult to suggest, without further information or observation, how much impact the sexual abuse has had on Molly. Therefore some assumptions will have to be made during formulation. It would be important to think about the context of the sexual abuse and also the developmental stage which normally occurs around age nine, as the abuse may have interfered with that development (Putnam, 2006). There are some indicators within her account that she has difficulty with sexual intimacy (reporting anxious thoughts about it "going too far" and feeling "dirty"), which are responses commonly reported by sexual abuse survivors (Sanderson, 2006). Pelvic pain and IBS are also commonly reported by sexual abuse and trauma survivors (Paras et al., 2009); IBS has been linked by some authors with chronic hyperarousal (Kendall-Tackett, 2000), and pain has been described as "procedural memory for the sensorimotor experiences of the trauma" (Scaer, 2014, p. 104), so we would see the physical symptoms as potentially linked to a trauma response within Molly.

Trauma is tracked in the present moment via autonomic nervous system (ANS) arousal. Some of Molly's currently reported difficulties, such as 'butterflies in the stomach', needing to go to the loo, difficulty sleeping, and shallow breathing, are indicative of ANS arousal in response to perceived threat (a trauma response). However, it should also be noted that the S/W character is also a trauma-based strategy and tends to have high ANS arousal in response to attachment based threat, so an observed high ANS arousal could be linked to character and/or the past abuse history. Central to BCP theory and practice is the 'Window of Tolerance' model of ANS dysregulation (Siegel, 1999), which proposes that between the extremes of hyperarousal and hypoarousal, there is a 'window' within which emotions and body sensations can be tolerated, and information can be processed and integrated with this experience. Animal defensive responses, such as 'fight', 'flight', 'freeze', 'submit', and 'attach' are mapped onto this model of autonomic arousal at the two extremes (Corrigan, Fisher, & Nutt, 2011). The model is utilised widely within BCP to track the client's autonomic arousal, with the aim of increasing their ability to be aware of their arousal patterns and triggers, and to ultimately be better able to regulate their arousal levels (Corrigan et al., 2011; Ogden, Minton, & Pain, 2006). Molly's ANS arousal would therefore be tracked during sessions, and this model discussed with her so she can start to mindfully track her own arousal levels and any triggers which may lead to hyper- or hypoarousal. We would also look for signs of dissociation occurring within the session or client report. There is little in the case description to suggest the presence of problematic dissociative experiences. However, we would continue to be vigilant for this and work with it using Sensorimotor Psychotherapy (Ogden & Fisher, 2014; Ogden et al., 2006) if it was present.

9.2.3 Present Moment Experience

When meeting with Molly, present moment to moment experience would be tracked and contact made with what is being experienced. From the case description there is little information about the 'core organisers' which Molly experiences during the therapeutic sessions. However, there are some interesting details which allow for supposition and inform the formulation below. Molly's anger with the therapist in the first session is initially surprising, as a predominant S/W presentation would suggest a more withdrawn presentation. The fact that she was angry could mean that this strategy is already softening, or that another strategy was dominant, or that a trauma response had been triggered within the session. This is discussed further below.

9.2.4 Initial Formulation

9.2.4.1 Developmental Issues–Attachment and Character

It is hypothesised that Molly demonstrates an insecure-avoidant primary attachment style, a presentation which is described by Ogden and colleagues (2006, p. 49; p. 55) in terms of a tendency to withdraw from others, preferring self-regulation, and to minimise attachment needs. There is a tendency to avoid expression of emotions, and an over-regulation of emotional responses. How this can present in the body is varied as some may present as quite rigid in muscle tone and may pull back from others, whereas some may have a more passive structure in their body. This is also similar in presentation and linked to the S/W character strategy, which will be discussed further.

Given our hypothesis discussed above, it is proposed that Molly's predominant character strategy is S/W, with elements of E/C, and we therefore formulate her case on this assumption while being open to acknowledging the presence of other strategies. As the case information also suggests that Molly's current difficulties may have traumatic roots, it is important to acknowledge a likely trauma background, which will interact with these character strategies. People who have the S/W strategy tend to be quite isolated, and to withdraw from or avoid social contact (Kurtz, 1990), as discussed above. Molly is single, lives alone, and tends not to socialise much as she finds large groups difficult. This may indicate a tendency to withdraw as she feels unwelcome in groups and may feel like a 'stranger in a strange and dangerous land' (Kurtz, 1990, p. 43) when in a group setting. She only felt able to socialise with her housemates when specifically asked to do so, as she did not wish to impose on the group. Molly also felt that she did not 'fit in' when working as a classroom assistant. There is further indication of this strategy where she feels 'stressed' and 'exposed' at university when having to take part in role plays, presentations, and class discussions, which would be particularly threatening to this character strategy which takes refuge in avoiding being seen. Molly does have one long term friend (Eve), but seems to also keep her at distance, talking to her on the phone once a week (although it is not clear whether Eve lives close enough to Molly for regular face to face contact). More recently it seemed like this strategy relaxed a little in relation to Amy, who began working at the library, and a brief friendship began to develop. However, when Molly thought she heard Amy making a comment about her, this would have felt threatening and triggered a return to her default way of being (withdrawing and avoiding). The same withdrawal and avoidance pattern emerged after her encounter with Jack. We would hypothesise that the S/W pattern would manifest in Molly's body with tension (often within the core) and, with trauma responses (ANS arousal) easily triggered, she may have a tendency in her body to pull away from contact with other people. Her body may physically hold the core belief around 'holding oneself together' via the tension and a 'holding in' pattern in the whole body. Core beliefs linking with this pattern might be around not belonging or being welcome, or the world not being safe, so it is likely that these beliefs would be present for Molly.

The childhood environment described is also consistent with a need for this adaptive strategy to be developed. Her home life is described as 'lacking warmth' and her parents living very separate lives within the same home. It is therefore unlikely that there was much emotional or physical contact between Molly and her parents, and it is likely that she would have had to learn to distance herself from people in order to cope with this environment. It is likely that she would have had many experiences of her emotional needs not being met, which would have left her having to manage these emotions, mainly by shutting them down and learning to manage them by herself. This would then be reflected in her body and muscular pattern, as her body organised itself around containing these emotions. The S/W strategy is often observed in the body as tension, tightness, and appearing to lack emotion and seeming 'cold' to other people (Kurtz, 1990). Fisher and Boreham (2014a) suggest that S/W is characterised by 'holding and tension' in the body and the person is 'internally frightened, extremely sensitive, often suspicious or on guard, finding it difficult to make contact because it feels as if the only safety is withdrawal far inside' (Fisher & Boreham, 2014b). Indeed, Cotter names this the "Hold Together" personality. A pattern of holding and tension is also likely to affect breathing, so Molly may display a pattern of shallow breathing as well. There may also be a startled or withdrawn look in the eyes (Cotter, 1996).

Emotions may be quite cut-off in someone who has a predominant S/W strategy, and this may be the case with Molly, as she has learnt to not display emotions or needs, because these were not recognised or accepted. This could be observed as tension in her jaw/mouth as she learnt as a child to hold in her emotions rather than to express them. The S/W strategy often withdraws internally into cognitions, and becomes very analytical, splitting off from emotional content. However, there are also various strengths in this strategy, one of which is creativity and analytical abilities, as people withdraw into a world of imagination, theory, analysis, and fantasy (Kurtz, 1990), and in certain circumstances these characteristics can be very useful.

Within therapy, Molly is described as appearing very tense and sitting very still and upright. The phrase 'pull/keep herself together' is mentioned three times and is likely to reflect a core belief which could be manifested in the body in a 'pulling in' around the central torso area. However, it is mentioned in the context of 'I *should* be able to pull myself together', which may mean that she is finding it difficult to continue with this strategy amongst her current difficulties.

During the first session, it is noted that her gaze fluctuated between the therapist and the door, which is suggestive that a 'flight' response had been triggered, and her body, via the ANS, had geared up to quickly leave the situation which was so anxiety provoking for her. We could theorise that the therapy setting is threatening or anxiety provoking because her S/W strategy would not want the therapist to 'see' or engage with her, and so this triggers her ANS into hyperarousal. She appears to manage this desire to leave and remains in the session; however, it could be hypothesised that by suppressing her body's 'flight' response, this leads to a 'fight' response being triggered. With the ANS arousal high, she may be outside of her window of tolerance and the anger, confrontational, and critical behaviour could therefore be a 'fight' response to the perceived threatening situation.

Other perhaps less dominant character strategies, which may be triggered by specific situations, are also indicated within the case description. We will briefly discuss Expressive Clinging (E/C) here as it appears particularly relevant to Molly's close relationships and her stay on the ward, and may be helpful to the formulation, both to understand her behaviour and predict how she may present at times in therapy. This strategy dramatises and amplifies events and feelings in order to gain attention and to maintain relationships. The desire is to avoid separation and utilises dramatisation to delay ending relationships or conversations (hence the 'clinging' part of the term), representing a need for love and attention which has not previously been received (Kurtz,

1990). There are some indications of this E/C strategy being present for Molly, as she is reported to have been seen as “controlling”, “emotionally demanding”, “overly emotional”, “clingy” and “dramatic” by others, particularly when a relationship is under threat of ending. On the ward, the nurses are reported to have experienced her as “histrionic”, and “attention seeking”, which also could have been due to the activation of the E/C strategy as she sought to gain attention from staff members. It is possible that the staff who felt they had established a positive relationship were able to meet some of her needs for attention and consideration, and therefore this strategy was not needed. As mentioned above, it is possible that Molly is pulled between her two main character strategies – one desiring separation and withdrawal to feel safe, the other desiring contact, and maintaining this through drama and ‘clinging’. This could therefore create quite a conflict within Molly, and be confusing to others as she exhibits seemingly contrasting behaviour at different times.

9.2.4.2 Trauma

Whilst there is less information about any traumatic effects of the sexual abuse, it is suggested that Molly has had particular difficulties in sexual intimacy, which we would suggest is linked to her past abuse history. Her reports of feeling “dirty” and worries about sexual intimacy “going too far” suggest that it continues to affect her. Within a body focused therapy it may be difficult for her to focus on her body because of what that might mean for her in relation to the past abuse. It is also possible, however, that she might be re-experiencing physical symptoms of trauma in her body, and may have difficulty regulating her nervous system and physiological arousal levels due to the remnants of past trauma. This might be related to the abuse in her past history, and may be particularly triggered when there is a perceived ‘threat’ of sexual intimacy. The level of trauma-related physiological arousal would be tracked within sessions, particularly when sexual relationships are discussed. It is likely that if unresolved trauma is held in the body then it would need to be processed as part of the therapeutic work.

The formulation would be held in mind whilst working with Molly, but is flexible and open to change depending on new information and insights that might emerge. In addition, the focus of each session would also be negotiated with Molly, and the therapist would have a ‘mini-formulation’ within each session about the current issue being addressed and the possibility of change within that issue.

9.2.5 Intervention Objectives

An essential element in body focused psychotherapy is establishing mindfulness (Kurtz, 1990). This is discussed with the client and taught from the beginning of therapy; the interventions require the client to be mindful (noticing their present moment experiences) rather than being 'hijacked' by the past experience being discussed (Ogden et al., 2006). One of the key differences about this therapy is that we are interested primarily in mindful observation of present moment experience when a difficulty from the past is being discussed. This enables dual awareness, rather than getting caught up in the past, and enables people to learn to stay within the window of tolerance during therapy in order to process past traumas (Fisher, 2011b; Ogden et al., 2006). From first meeting the client, the therapist also engages in mindful tracking (observing) of what the client experiences in the body as we assess how they organise experience through the core elements of body sensation, movement, sensory perception, cognition, and emotion (Kurtz, 1990), and how cognitions and emotions are experienced in the body. The therapist makes 'contact' with what they notice, through the use of contact statements (Kurtz, 1990), such as: 'As you say those words, your leg starts to shake'. The therapist also engages in 'body reading', looking for procedurally learnt and long standing physical and postural tendencies that may reflect long held beliefs and patterns of emotion, attachment, and strategies of character (Ogden et al., 2006). Within mindfulness, an 'experimental attitude' is fostered, and a variety of experiments are used to explore and work with key issues (Kurtz, 1990). For example, the client might be asked to 'notice what happens when...' the therapist or client does or says something (Kurtz, 1990). Objectives of intervention and the process of therapy depend on whether there is a traumatic or developmental focus for the session; we will comment on both here given that both appear relevant in Molly's case.

9.2.5.1 Trauma

Similar to other trauma-focussed therapies, BCP takes a three-phased approach to treatment. Ogden et al. (2006) label these phases as: (1) Developing Somatic Resources for Stabilization; (2) Processing Traumatic Memory and Restoring Acts of Triumph; and (3) Integration and Success in Normal Life. The aim is to create stability, resources, increase the ability to regulate arousal, and stay within the window of tolerance before traumatic memories are accessed and processed through the body. During Sensorimotor Psychotherapy for trauma, the patient learns to regulate their autonomic arousal and to gain more control over their response to trauma-related stimuli. They also gain greater understanding of how recalling trauma affects their current experience of their body, thoughts, and emotions, and to notice these in the present without judging or interpreting them. In addition, they learn to discriminate more clearly between past and present experience, facilitating an ability to recall the traumatic event without feeling overwhelmed, leading to a sense of the event as being "finally over" (Fisher, 2011b, p. 174).

9.2.5.2 Development & Attachment

The objectives for developmental work are similar in that they are aimed at "addressing the bodily and autonomic symptoms of ... attachment-related disorders, as well as the cognitive-emotional aspects" (Fisher, 2011a, p. 101). For clients with an insecure-avoidant attachment, or S/W strategy, the therapeutic objectives are to increase the ability to engage with others when their arousal is at a higher level than they have previously been able to cope with. Ogden et al. (2006) state that to "practice managing this higher arousal state during interpersonal interaction fosters a wider window of tolerance" (p. 58), acknowledging that a slow paced approach is needed to avoid psychological and physical defences being triggered. For Molly, this would mean that through the process of therapy we would aim to explore and create resources to enable her to tolerate being in social situations more, and feel less like she has to withdraw from them. This would work directly with long held patterns related to her predominant attachment/character style.

The framework for a developmental session is presented in Kurtz (1990, pp. 72-73). Within the therapeutic relationship, mindfulness is established, and a 'frame' (focus) for the session created as experience is evoked: "thoughts, feelings, images, memories, sensations, tensions, impulses, and the emergence of the child" (p.72). A variety of techniques can be used to 'access and deepen into the experience', and then the session moves into 'state-specific processing', where the therapist accesses core material through the body and other core organisers, working with the child state and with strong emotions (which Kurtz sometimes calls 'Riding the Rapids'). The aim is to use technique to "create the experience that wants to happen" (Kurtz, 1990, p. 72), following which the client experiences a transformation in their body, emotions and/or beliefs. This new experience is then integrated through the body, cognition, and emotion, and ends with 'completion' (see below for specific examples of techniques).

In Molly's case we may work with the trauma process first, as it is likely that she may need to learn to regulate her arousal and stay within the window of tolerance to even enable her to engage with the therapeutic process. We would therefore start with resource-building and stabilisation before working on any traumatic issues from the past abuse. The work with attachment/developmental patterns and character strategies may be interspersed with the trauma work, where appropriate, depending on what is triggered for her, or in the field, at each session.

It is an anticipated part of the process that barriers will emerge during therapy, and indeed Kurtz (1990) recognises a number of possible points at which this may happen. He names these "insight, response, nourishment and completion barriers" (p.170). The ways these barriers emerge are strongly linked to long-held patterns based on early attachments and experiences, and they are acknowledged and worked with as part of the therapy.

It is also anticipated that Molly may have a 'phobia of therapy and the therapist' (Ogden et al., 2006; Steele, van der Hart, & Nijenhuis, 2001) which would need initial attention. With her avoidant attachment pattern, it may feel very threatening to engage with another person in such an intimate way, and it may take a while to build a therapeutic relationship with her for this reason. It may be useful to use experiments around proximity to help her to explore this further (see below).

Mindful observation, therapist tracking, and client report are the main within-session measure of whether these objectives are being achieved. In addition, there may be a transformation which is reached but needs integrating into the client's life to show whether the process has been effective. Therefore, therapist and client might agree a way for the client to test something out in their life between sessions. Client reports of improvement in their life, their body, cognitions, and emotions are the main ways of assessing therapy progress and effectiveness. In trauma work we would look for less autonomic arousal in relation to the trauma, whereas in developmental work we would look for relaxation of character strategy and therefore greater freedom to act with more choice within their life.

9.2.6 Intervention Plan

Initial sessions would focus on resource building and stabilisation, and would involve considerable psychoeducation about the nature of trauma, the window of tolerance, and how the body is involved in this. Therapist and client would track the body and how it participates in discussion about current and past issues. Mindfulness skills would also be a focus of initial sessions. The therapist should also pay attention to their own physiological arousal levels in sessions in response to the client, and any somatic transference/countertransference which is experienced (Ogden et al., 2006; Rothschild & Rand, 2006). Whilst we would work in therapy with any of Molly's character strategies that emerged during the process, we will focus here on S/W for clarity and to demonstrate some of the possible interventions we would consider.

In working with the 'phobia of the therapist and therapy', experiments using proximity may be helpful. Molly, whilst being mindful, would be asked to observe what happens in her body and other core organisers when physical proximity to the therapist is changed; for example, the therapist moving one step closer or further away from her. In this way, we can explore the body's reaction to proximity to others, and how this is also experienced in her emotions and beliefs. Finding a distance from which Molly feels comfortable undertaking therapy will help with the 'interactive regulation' (Ogden et al., 2006, pp. 58-59; pp. 214-216) of her nervous system, and enable her to stay within the window of tolerance in therapy sessions. It would also enable study of her S/W character strategy, acknowledging where her boundaries lie, and enabling work with them, to help her to tolerate closer proximity and the higher arousal that creates, giving her the opportunity to explore and test this out in therapy before trying it out in situations in her life.

The therapist would need to be mindful of the predominant S/W strategy and adjust their style accordingly; for example, an over empathic therapist may drive an

S/W client to withdraw. It is important to also respect the positive aspects which the character strategy brings and how this has helped the person to survive to this point in time. Molly will have a strong preference for 'auto regulation' (i.e., regulating her own feelings and body as opposed to someone else helping her to do this) and so early experiments in therapy may involve seeing whether she can tolerate any 'interactive regulation' for even a moment (Ogden et al., 2006, pp. 58-59).

At each session, the focus for the session will be agreed, and the therapist would be aware of whether it is likely to have a trauma or developmental focus.

9.2.6.1 Trauma

Assuming that trauma work is needed, we would begin by developing somatic resources to enable stabilisation and increased ability to regulate body and emotions. An initial aim is to build upon and develop existing resources which are held within the body. This might arise from the therapist noticing a movement which occurs when a particularly resourceful belief is mentioned, for example, or to strengthen the client's ability to say 'no' (Ogden et al., 2006). The movement might be an indication of a resource held within the body which the therapist would draw attention to and strengthen. The therapist would look for hints of somatic resources within Molly's presentation, and build upon what emerges. There could also be experiments around posture and movement; for example, if Molly presents as very tense and 'upright', then she might be encouraged to experiment with movement or relaxing tension, and noticing what happens as she does this. Development of other somatic resources might involve centering exercises (e.g., the client putting a hand on the core and a hand on the heart), grounding (e.g., increasing awareness of the feet on the floor, or the body supported by the chair), breath work (e.g., careful awareness of how the client tends to breathe, and experiments with changing these patterns to regulate arousal), and boundary work (e.g., experiments to enable the client to experience their personal boundaries) (Fisher, 1999; Ogden et al., 2006, pp. 224-223). These somatic resources are practiced and strengthened, then applied to 'future templates' (imagining future challenging situations), and then on into the client's life (Ogden et al., 2006, p. 233).

If trauma responses are still held in the body, or the body is holding an active defence that wanted to happen at the time but could not, then sessions would involve sensorimotor processing of the traumatic experience during the second phase of therapy, or work around reinstating an active defence (Ogden et al., 2006). Sensorimotor Psychotherapy offers one method of processing, called sensorimotor sequencing (described in Ogden et al., 2006, p. 253). Other body focused options for processing trauma are also presented by Levine's (1997) somatic experiencing therapy, or Rothschild's (2000) somatic trauma therapy.

9.2.6.2 Development, Attachment, and Character

Developmental sessions would take the form suggested by Kurtz (1990), as presented above. Within this overall structure, it would enable work on the key early memories that led to the formation of core beliefs, as the child 'map maker' made sense of how to manoeuvre through the social and physical world (Kurtz, 1990). These core beliefs can be accessed in a number of ways, but a key technique is "going for meaning" (Kurtz, 1990), where core beliefs are expressed in the form of bodily tension, gestures, movements etc. Kurtz (1990, p. 141) describes this technique, where tension in the body is noticed, emphasised, and mindfully observed in detail. The therapist then asks questions such as "If this tension could speak, what would it say?" or "What are you saying with your body when you tense that way?" (Kurtz, 1990). In this way, core beliefs and meanings are discovered, accessing them via the body.

Experiments such as "Taking Over" might also be used. This is where the therapist takes over something that the client procedurally does, to allow the client to experience something different. For example, if Molly was hyper-vigilant and constantly watching the door, the therapist could take that over for her (i.e., watch the door), allowing Molly more freedom to look around the room and ground herself within the environment. If there is a pattern of tension in the body, the therapist might also "take over" this for the client as an experiment (Kurtz, 1990).

Probes might also be used as an experiment during different parts of the process (Rothschild, 2000). Verbal probes are words which are said by the therapist to the client (usually relating to a missing experience that the client has never had), where the client is asked to mindfully observe their response to the words being said, so that they respond rather than react (Kurtz, 1990). A probe which is often used for an S/W strategy is: "You're welcome here" (Kurtz, 1990), which would likely be an appropriate experiment for Molly given the formulation. She would be asked to notice what happens when she hears those words, in relation to all of the core organisers (body sensation, five senses, movement, thoughts, and emotions) and report what she notices. A reaction is expected, such as a bodily or emotional response, or a thought such as: "I'm not". Sometimes a probe is used as a way to access and work with a past memory – to evoke an experience to work with at a deeper level. It is quite possible that using this probe with Molly might lead her to access a memory of not feeling welcome, perhaps in a situation from her early childhood. As the early childhood memory is likely to be more linked to 'core material', we would work with that memory through the process described by Kurtz (1990): accessing the core material and working with the child state of consciousness, accessing strong emotions and allowing them to emerge, aiming to create the experience that 'wants to happen'. Kurtz is clear that the adult always remains part of this process as dual awareness is maintained:

"The child and its experiences built the world view and the self-image. The child was the map maker. So, in contacting and working with the child, you have the possibility of changing those maps and the person who is now using them. By just being there with that child, by talking to it and holding it, and explaining things, by being careful and concerned and patient, just by doing that you change the way that child feels about itself and the world. And in doing that, you can change the adult, too" (Kurtz, 1990, p. 133).

In Molly's case the missing experience might be to truly feel welcome, and for her child parts to have the experience of feeling welcome too, aiming to create a shift in her beliefs and emotions. However, the process is creative and can utilise various techniques as appropriate; it is therefore difficult to predict exactly what might emerge during therapy with Molly, and which specific techniques might be used, without further therapeutic interaction with Molly herself. Other possibilities are the use of physical experiments (Ogden et al., 2006, p. 49) and 'Magical Stranger' (Kurtz, 1990) among others.

In summary, BCP offers a holistic way of formulating and intervening with individuals, considering bodily experience (alongside cognitions and emotions) as central to understanding a client's difficulties. It is a creative, flexible way of working that is informed by the client's needs at each session. However, this in itself makes BCP a difficult intervention to research in a randomised way, and the challenges of establishing its effectiveness remain.

David M Gresswell

9.3 BCP Formulation: Critical Commentary

In considering this chapter it is very difficult to get to any underlying theory on which the approach is based. Very early on, the authors make the point that the fundamental defining principle of BCP is that we are "bodies"; however, they then concede that most other modern psychological theories agree with this perspective. Furthermore they also rapidly acknowledge that BCP is primarily a repertoire of techniques drawing on a range of influences: Clearly this is an unfortunate position from which to undertake a formulation. Indeed all the more unfortunate in that a coherent account of the phenomenology of human emotional experience also seems to be missing from the approach. Instead, the focus is on physical habits, mannerisms, and "character strategies" (character strategies are essentially a form of personality typology involving eight different ways of relating to the world that are at least "functionally rather than pathologically" labelled). The authors admit that there is very little evidence to support the validity, utility, or efficacy of any of this but attempt to defend their stance by stating that the outcomes BCP practitioners are interested in are "difficult to put into words".

Despite all this, the authors' "initial hypothesis" is that Molly's current issues are derived from the "character strategies" that she acquired in early childhood and consolidated thereafter. The character strategies identified essentially describe Molly's avoidance and clinginess, and the approach/avoidance conflict that inevitably arises from these two competing social strategies. The authors also consider the possibility of Molly's problems having "traumatic roots" (the alleged sexual abuse at the age of 9 years old – the nature of which is currently unknown) and make "assumptions" that this experience has contributed to Molly's current difficulties with sexual intimacy. At one level, this is a reasonable assumption. However, in practice, when considering the role of the alleged trauma, the focus on the body "in the present moment" causes at least two problems which potentially impair the development of a comprehensive formulation: Firstly, given Molly's account of a neglectful childhood, she may have been particularly vulnerable to being targeted by others for abuse (as noted above, we do not know anything about the nature of the alleged abuse); secondly, it would imply that the adult relationship/sexual conflicts she reports were not the primary causes of the sexual problems she describes in adulthood. The BCP approach to formulation does not appear to have the flexibility to accommodate these alternative possibilities.

In practice, within the main formulation section, the authors initially put BCP to one side and begin with attachment theory. They describe how an "insecure avoidant attachment style" will be expressed in terms of either a "quite rigid muscle tone" and associated withdrawal or "more passive structures" – such variability in expression, with potential for quite disparate presentations, would presumably make it difficult to interpret the individual's responses. The authors nevertheless diagnose a primary "Sensitive/Withdrawn" character strategy with elements of an "Expressive/Clinging" (E/C) character strategy. These diagnoses then struggle to account for observable but, from the perspective of BCP at least, conflicting behaviours, such as Molly "relaxing" her character strategies when she meets Amy (at work), and indeed her anger directed at the therapist. Faced with this difficulty, the authors simply change their primary model/terminology and suggest that Molly's "body may physically hold" core beliefs that account for the conflicting observations. Various other descriptions of Molly's posture follow before the authors move on to talk about possible interventions. It is unclear how Molly's body (as opposed to Molly) can hold or express a core belief.

With respect to intervention the authors propose that a "key difference" between BCP and other therapies is focus on "in the moment experience of when a difficulty from the past is being discussed" which enables the client to "learn to stay within a window of tolerance" – essentially a moderate, tolerable level of physiological arousal. Other intervention strategies include focussing on the "autonomic symptoms" of the purported underlying attachment disorder. However, in essence, the process of intervention described here primarily involves an unstructured desensitisation/exposure programme in which attention is drawn to various physical habits and responses. Whether Molly's body, her brain, or Molly herself is being affected by all this counter conditioning seems largely irrelevant for the practical purposes of BCP – although, seemingly at random, the authors finally suggest that, from a BCP perspective, asking Molly a series of questions around whether she "feels welcome" might be helpful.

Given all of the above it is difficult to see what, if anything, BCP can contribute to either a formulation or intervention that other approaches do not do better, other than increasing client and therapist attention on physical signs of distress. The underlying BCP approach to formulation as articulated here seems to be an eclectic and rather uncritical brew, drawing on a little attachment theory, a measure of personality diagnosis, and a pinch of cognitive structuralism. All these ingredients can be found in other psychological models, some of which also have an evidence-base. Similarly, the suggested BCP intervention strategies also draw on an assorted range of sources (but would seem in essence to be reducible to unstructured covert and overt counter conditioning paradigms). On balance, it would therefore seem that BCP has more in common with so-called integrative approaches, than with evidence-based, theoretically driven approaches. Consequently, I would suggest that clinicians give preference to familiarising themselves with a more coherent and empirically-supported model of human action/intervention, whilst bearing in mind the common sense observation that we should attend to what our clients do as well as what they say.

Rachel Sabin-Farrell & Roger Bretherton

9.4 Author response

Writing about BCP in a volume explicitly dedicated to psychological formulation is problematic to say the least. In recent times, it is largely the advocates of behavioural therapies who have most emphasised the notion of formulation, whereas body psychotherapy prefers to explain its therapeutic rationale without using the term formulation at all. Writing from a body perspective in the present volume therefore feels somewhat like playing to an away crowd. And inevitably, in response, the author of the critical commentary musters the stridency that comes from standing on familiar ground.

Primarily, it is important to address the accusation of theoretical inconsistency. The critical commentary suggests that BCP draws on an inadequately bolted together set of theories and techniques. It is asserted that we draw on personality type, then shift to attachment theory, then leap on cognitive constructionism. Nothing could be further from the truth of BCP in practice.

It is true that BCP does draw on a wide range of psychological theory. This is one of its strengths. In a brief chapter it is difficult to elaborate the points of integration between developmental neuropsychology, attachment theory, gestalt psychotherapy, cognitive-behavioural theory, and the numerous other ingredients that make up the consistent flavour of BCP. The task is made more difficult by the fact that many of these conceptual underpinnings are not shared by other contributors to this volume. To convince an audience of newcomers to the approach, more explanation is needed than can be allowed here.

This theoretical diversity however, is not a weakness of BCP, but rather its strength. One of the central commitments of the body centred approach is *holism*: the view that everything in the human body, mind, and context connect together and influence one another. All formulations by definition take some small slither of this whole for the purposes of making a beneficial intervention, but no formulation captures the entire ecology of the presenting client and her problem. BCP as an approach is therefore deeply committed to not confusing the map with the territory. Just as geographically accurate maps are arrived at through numerous techniques of photography, surveillance, observation, and sampling, so too are accurate views of the clinical situation derived from numerous perspectives, none of which can claim to be the whole truth.

BCP essentially is a critique of the very notion of formulation. The body from this perspective *is* the formulation: the structural expression of the client's resources and stresses that, if attended to carefully, directs therapeutic intervention. Far from being a string of boxes and arrows in the therapist's head, the formulation is the bones and sinew of the client's body, from which the therapist develops intervention based on the client's experience as well as theory. It is not a dogmatic formula to be defended, but a living phenomenon to be explored. This lends BCP a singular advantage over the more abstruse constructions of behavioural theory – the advantage of being *real* and centred upon present moment phenomena.

References

Campbell, P. A., & McMahon, E. M. (1997). *Bio-spirituality: Focusing as a way to grow*. Chicago: Loyola Press.

Carroll, R. (2003). At the border between chaos and order": What psychotherapy and neuroscience have in common. In J. Corrigall & H. Wilkinson (Eds.), *Revolutionary connections: Psychotherapy and neuroscience* (pp. 191-211). London: Karnac.

Corrigan, F. M., Fisher, J. J., & Nutt, D. J. (2011). Autonomic dysregulation and the Window of Tolerance model of the effects of complex emotional trauma. *Journal of Psychopharmacology, 25*(1), 17-25.

Cotter, S. (1996). Using bioenergetics to develop managers: Ten years of practical application of body-mind psychology with over a thousand managers at Cranfield University. *Journal of Management Development, 15*(3), 8-16.

Dinas, S. (2012). *The Body In Therapy: Experiences of Sensorimotor Psychotherapy*. University of Nottingham. Unpublished Doctoral Thesis.

Fisher, J. (1999). The work of stabilization in trauma treatment. *Trauma Center Lecture Series, Boston, Massachusetts*.

Fisher, J. (2011a). Attachment as a Sensorimotor Experience: The Use of Sensorimotor Psychotherapy. *Attachment: New Directions in Psychotherapy and Relational Psychoanalysis, 5*(2), 99-107.

Fisher, J. (2011b). Sensorimotor approaches to trauma treatment. *Advances in Psychiatric Treatment, 17*(3), 171-177.

Fisher, J., & Boreham, P. (2014a). 'Character strategies' (Part One) – Dr Janina Fisher's insights. Retrieved from http://www.khironhouse.com/blog/character-strategies-dr-janina-fishers-insights/

Fisher, J., & Boreham, P. (2014b). Character Strategies (Part Two) – 'Sensitive-Withdrawn' And 'Sensitive-Emotional' – Dr Janina Fisher's insights. Retrieved from http://www.khironhouse.com/blog/character-strategies-dr-janina-fishers-insights/

Fisher, J., & Ogden, P. (2009). Sensorimotor psychotherapy. In C. A. Courtois & J. D. Ford (Eds.), *Treating complex traumatic stress disorders: An evidence-based guide* (pp. 312-328). New York: The Guilford Press.

Friedman, N. (2007). *Focusing-Oriented Therapy: (Fot)*. Lincoln: iUniverse.

Gendlin, E. T. (2003). *Focusing: How To Gain Direct Access To Your Body's Knowledge*. London: Random House.

Gerhardt, S. (2006). Why love matters: How affection shapes a baby's brain. *Infant Observation, 9*(3), 305-309.

Glazer, R., & Friedman, H. (2009). The Construct Validity of the Bioenergetic–Analytic Character Typology: A Multi-Method Investigation of a Humanistic Approach to Personality. *The Humanistic Psychologist, 37*(1), 24-48.

Johnson, S. M. (1994). *Character styles*. New York: Norton.

Keleman, S. (1981). *Your Body Speaks Its Mind*. Berkeley: Center Press.

Kendall-Tackett, K. A. (2000). Physiological correlates of childhood abuse: chronic hyperarousal in PTSD, depression, and irritable bowel syndrome. *Child Abuse & Neglect, 24*(6), 799-810.

Kepner, J. I. (1987). *Body process: Working with the body in psychotherapy*. San Francisco: Jossey-Bass.

Kurtz, R. (1990). *Body-centered Psychotherapy: The Hakomi Method*. Mendocino, CA: LifeRhythm.

Langmuir, J. I., Kirsh, S. G., & Classen, C. C. (2012). A pilot study of body-oriented group psychotherapy: Adapting sensorimotor psychotherapy for the group treatment of trauma. *Psychological Trauma: Theory, Research, Practice, and Policy, 4*(2), 214-220.

Lanius, R., Lanius, U., Fisher, J., & Ogden, P. (2006). Psychological trauma and the brain: Towards a neurobiological treatment model. In P. Ogden, K. Minton & C. Pain (Eds.), *Trauma and the body: A sensorimotor approach to psychotherapy* (pp. 139-161). New York: Norton.

Levine, P. A. (1997). *Waking the tiger: Healing trauma: The innate capacity to transform overwhelming experiences*. Berkeley: North Atlantic Books.

Lowen, A. (1975). *Bioenergetics*. London: Penguin.

Marcel, G. (1964). *Creative fidelity* (R. Rosthal, Trans.). New York: Fordham University Press.

Ogden, P., & Fisher, J. (2014). *Sensorimotor psychotherapy: Interventions for trauma and attachment*. New York, NY: Norton.

Ogden, P., Minton, K., & Pain, C. (2006). *Trauma and the Body: A Sensorimotor Approach to Psychotherapy (Norton Series on Interpersonal Neurobiology)*. New York: W. W. Norton.

Padesky, C. A., & Greenberger, D. (1995). *Clinician's guide to mind over mood*. London: Guilford Press.

Paras, M. L., Murad, M. H., Chen, L. P., Goranson, E. N., Sattler, A. L., Colbenson, K. M., . . . Zirakzadeh, A. (2009). Sexual abuse and lifetime diagnosis of somatic disorders: a systematic review and meta-analysis. *JAMA, 302*(5), 550-561.

Putnam, F. W. (2006). The impact of trauma on child development. *Juvenile and Family Court Journal, 57*(1), 1-11.

Reich, W. (1980). *Character analysis*. London: Macmillan.

Rothschild, B. (2000). *The body remembers: The psychophysiology of trauma and trauma treatment*. New York: WW Norton & Company.

Rothschild, B. (2003). *The Body Remembers Casebook: Unifying Methods and Models in the Treatment of Trauma and PTSD*. New York: W.W. Norton.

Rothschild, B., & Rand, M. (2006). Help for the helper: Self-care strategies for managing burnout and stress. *New York & London: WW Norton & Company*.

Sanderson, C. (2006). *Counselling Adult Survivors of Child Sexual Abuse*. London: J. Kingsley.

Scaer, R. (2014). *The Body Bears the Burden: Trauma, Dissociation, and Disease*. New York: Routledge.
Schore, A. N. (2003). *Affect Regulation and the Repair of the Self (Norton Series on Interpersonal Neurobiology)* (Vol. 2). New York: WW Norton & Company.
Shapiro, F. (2001). *Eye Movement Desensitization and Reprocessing: Basic Principles, Protocols, and Procedures*. New York: Guilford Press.
Siegel, D. J. (1999). *The developing mind*. New York: Guilford Press.
Siegel, D. J. (2010). *Mindsight: The new science of personal transformation*. Oxford: One World.
Solomon, M., & Siegel, D. J. (2003). *Healing Trauma: Attachment, Mind, Body and Brain (Norton Series on Interpersonal Neurobiology)*. New York: WW Norton & Company.
Steele, K., van der Hart, O., & Nijenhuis, E. R. (2001). Dependency in the treatment of complex posttraumatic stress disorder and dissociative disorders. *Journal of Trauma & Dissociation, 2*(4), 79-116.
Totton, N. (2003). *Body psychotherapy: An introduction*. Maidenhead: Open University.
van der Kolk, B. (1996). The body keeps the score: approaches to the psychobiology of posttraumatic stress disorder. In B A van der Kolk, A. C. McFarlane & L. Weisaeth (Eds.), *Traumatic Stress: The Effects of Overwhelming Experience on Mind* (pp. 214-241). New York: Guilford.
van der Kolk, B. (2014). *The Body Keeps the Score: Mind, Brain and Body in the Transformation of Trauma*. London: Penguin Books Limited.
Yalom, I. D. (2009). *The Gift of Therapy: Reflections on Being a Therapist*. London: Piatkus.
Young, C. (2006). One hundred and fifty years on: The history, significance and scope of body psychotherapy today. *Body, Movement and Dance in Psychotherapy, 1*(1), 17-28.

Vanessa Dale-Hewitt & Chris Irons

10 Compassion Focused Therapy

Compassion Focused Therapy (CFT) is an integrated and multifaceted approach to working with individuals experiencing psychological and emotional distress (Gale, Gilbert, Read, & Goss, 2014; Gilbert, 2010; Gilbert & Irons, 2005). It has been described as part of the growing movement in Cognitive-Behavioural Therapy (CBT) which embraces compassion, mindfulness, imagery, and eastern philosophies as integral parts of psychological therapy (Gale et al., 2014; Gilbert, 2009a, 2014). Although sharing some similar principles with CBT (Westbrook, Kennerley, & Kirk, 2011), CFT differs in its philosophical underpinnings, understanding of psychological difficulties, and technical application. CFT aims to help people regulate affect and distress, and alleviate suffering, through the cultivation of compassion (Gilbert, 2010).

10.1 Historical Origins of Compassion Focused Therapy

CFT was developed by Paul Gilbert for people with complex and chronic mental health problems who were struggling to make progress in standard therapies (Gilbert, 2009a). Many of these people presented with high levels of shame and self-criticism, and had early life experiences characterised by high levels of threat (e.g., abuse, criticism, neglect) or the absence of care, affection, and love. Gilbert found that in using standard therapies (e.g., CBT), clients would report: "I know what you're saying, and I can see rationally that it wasn't my fault that I was abused, but I still feel like it was and that there's something wrong with me". This has been described as the head-heart lag, cognition-emotion mismatch, or rational emotional dissociation (Stott, 2007).

As Gilbert explored this experience with his clients, he recognised that, whilst many were able to generate helpful and evidence-based alternative thoughts in a standard cognitive way, the emotional tone of these new thoughts was often laced with a variety of negative emotions and feelings, such as anger, contempt, disappointment, or coldness. What also emerged was that, when asked to generate a more caring, warm, and compassionate feeling to go alongside the alternative thoughts, many clients found this very difficult, scary, or aversive. So, CFT developed initially as a way to help clients practice generating a certain type of positive emotional tone (e.g., in their tone of voice) that is rooted in a certain type of affiliative positive affect.

10.2 Theoretical Underpinnings and Central Tenets

CFT is grounded in a broad scientific literature and research base, and guided by findings from evolutionary, developmental, attachment, neuroscience, neurophysiological, and social psychological literatures. It also draws upon ideas from Buddhist philosophy and practice. There are a number of key theoretical ideas that underpin the approach:

10.2.1 Principle 1: Our Complex Minds and Motives Emerge from Evolutionary Processes

As an evolutionary psychology-informed approach, CFT suggests that, as part of the 'flow of life', humans evolved via the mammalian and then primate lines, and consequently share similar *motives* (e.g., to seek status, to form attachments, to nurture our children), *behavioural responses* (e.g., fight, flight, submission), and *basic emotions* (e.g., anger, anxiety, disgust). These are referred to as 'old brain' abilities. However, approximately two million years ago, pre-human ancestors began to evolve a range of new cognitive competencies linked to capacities for inductive and deductive reasoning, imagination, and anticipation, along with a capacity for complex self-monitoring and self-identity. Consequently, unlike other primates (as far as we know), we can anticipate things that haven't happened yet, ruminate about the past, and imagine various real and fantastic scenarios. Unfortunately, whilst evolution brings a variety of adaptive advantages, it does so via trade-offs. The way our minds have evolved has left them very 'tricky', with built in non-rational glitches which are vulnerable to unhelpful feedback loops (Gilbert, 1998). Examples can help clients understand this phenomenon, and a commonly used example in CFT is to consider a zebra running away from a lion. Once the zebra gets away, and the stimulus is no longer present in the olfactory visual or auditory domains (and nothing threatening remains), it will calm down relatively quickly. In contrast, a human would obviously be relieved to escape the clutches of a lion, but can recreate the stimulus profile in their own heads and imagine what might have happened if they had been caught (e.g., the lion eating them alive) or worry that the lion might come back. These processes will thus continually stimulate old brain emotions (e.g., anxiety) and defensive responses (e.g., flight, avoidance). Because we have a 'new' brain, we can bring threat stimuli that were once external 'inside the head', keeping them going even in the absence of an actual, current threat. Our old and new brain can get in to 'loops' that are not our fault (see Fig. 10.1). The key thing is that these loops can cause and drive much distress for people, and understanding the nature of these loops for our clients – and that these processes are not their fault – can be an important insight in CFT – a first step in formulation.

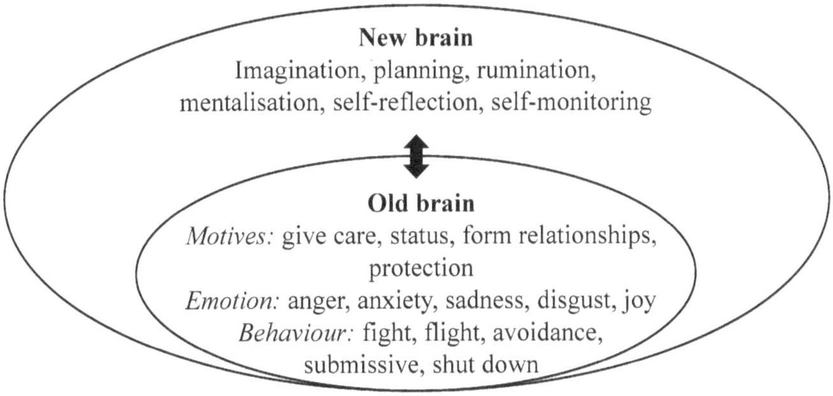

Figure 10.1: Old Brain/New Brain Interaction (adapted from Gilbert & Choden, 2013)

10.2.2 Principle 2: Our Sense of 'Self' is a Product of Our Genes and Socio-cultural Experiences

It is useful to help clients understand how our sense of 'self' emerges in the interaction between our evolved, genetically shaped minds and our social circumstances. Many of our clients have a sense of self – which often they describe in highly negative, denigratory terms – as somehow fixed or immutable; the 'I was born bad and defective' sense of self. However, we do not choose our genes, and for the most part, do not choose the types of experiences we have or social circumstances of our life (particularly in early life). Research has shown that our minds are highly plastic, as are our phenotypes (Belsky & Pluess, 2009), and scientific developments in understanding gene-environment interactions, including the study of behavioural epigenetics (e.g., Masterpasqua, 2009), are further contributing to our understanding that 'this version' of all of us is just one possible version of what might have been, given different genes and experiences. We ask our clients to imagine if we, as a therapist, had been abducted as a three-day old child by members of a violent drug gang. Here, clients are invited to imagine how the therapist might have been different if that had happened, how they might be more prone to certain emotions (e.g., anger), behaviours (e.g., aggression and violence) and types of relationship (e.g., mistrusting, abusive). These are not things that we ever wanted, but rather, emergent, phenotypic variations due to the interaction of our genes and experiences. There are a wide variety of different versions of us that may currently lie dormant, or could be shaped up with different experiences in the future. Therapy of course is one such experience that might help to bring a different version of self to the fore.

10.2.3 Principle 3: We Have Evolved Three Basic Emotion-regulation Systems

A key tenet of the model is developing an understanding of our basic evolved emotion systems and how they are balanced for our clients (see Fig. 10.2). Derived from the work of Panksepp (1998) and Depue and Morrone-Strupinsky (2005), CFT uses a simplified model of functional emotions in which we suggest that there are three basic emotion regulation systems:

The threat and self-protection system. This system evolved to help animals detect and respond to threats to themselves, but also important others (e.g., their offspring). To help in this process, this system utilises various brain systems (e.g., amygdala) and brain-body hormonal stress responses (the hypothalamic-pituitary-adrenal axis) to activate ancient behavioural responses (e.g., freeze, flight, fight, submission) and threat-based emotions (e.g., anger, anxiety, disgust) to help us manage threat and harm. Cognitive functioning under threat system activation often works on a 'better safe than sorry' basis, naturally biasing thinking and narrowing attention.

The drive seeking system. This system evolved to help animals seek out, pursue, and acquire important resources. This can include pursuing and acquiring important things like food, territory, and reproduction opportunities, along with social drives and rewards, for example, social approval, status, and power. It is a highly activating system, giving us bursts of energy that move us towards goals, and leaves us with certain types of positive feelings (joy, elation) when we have achieved them.

The contentment and soothing-affiliative system. When they are not managing threats, nor pursuing resources, it is important for animals to rest and recover. Sometimes known as the 'rest and digest' system, this affect regulation system is associated with a variety of lower energy positive emotions such as calmness, safeness, and contentment. It is linked to activation of the parasympathetic nervous system and vagus nerve (Porges, 2009) and to the neurohormones oxytocin and endorphin, and appears to have a naturally regulating effect on the threat system (e.g., Carter, 2014).

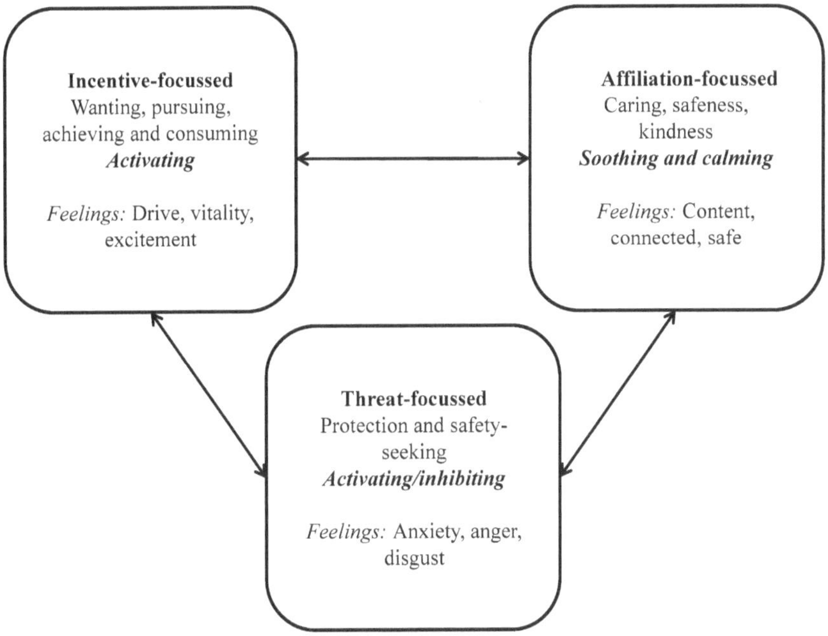

Figure 10.2: Our emotional regulation systems (adapted from Gilbert, 2009a)

10.2.4 Principle 4: Bringing Our Emotion-regulation Systems Into Balance Increases Well-being

CFT is concerned with the functioning of all three systems, but, in particular, the functioning and development of (or, in many cases, *block to*) the soothing-affiliative system. Mammals – and humans in particular – have evolved to be highly in need of, and responsive to, affiliative relationships and signals of care and affection (Carter, 2014). The experience of care and affiliative relationships impacts on a variety of threat-based physiological systems (e.g., Cozolino, 2007), genetic expression (Belsky & Pluess, 2009), and the way that we relate to ourselves and others (e.g., attachment theory; Bowlby, 1969).

10.3 What is Compassion?

Emerging initially out of parent-child mammalian dyads, the capacity to care for our young, the elderly, and for each other, is thought to have been a key behaviour in the success of mammals, including humans. Here, various qualities of caring and affiliation helped to facilitate these abilities, and out of these attributes emerged the more complex psychological process of compassion. CFT uses an adapted version of a common definition of compassion: “a sensitivity to the suffering of self and others (and the causes of that suffering) with a deep commitment to relieve it, prevent it from returning, and promote wellbeing.”

From a CFT perspective, this definition holds two different psychologies: (1) the attributes and capacity to be sensitive towards and engage with distress and suffering; and (2) the motivation and skill to try and alleviate suffering, prevent it from returning, and cultivate wellbeing. These two psychologies are represented in Figure 10.3, in which the inner circle indicates some of the key attributes of compassion that help us to engage distress (first psychology), and the outer circle the skills and interventions – as part of a multimodal therapy – that help to alleviate suffering (second psychology).

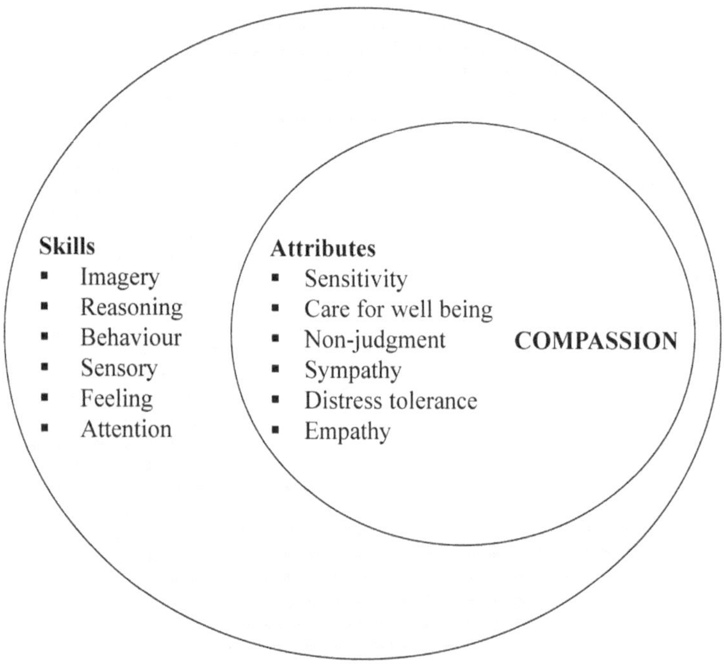

Figure 10.3: Compassion Attributes and Skills (adapted from Gilbert, 2009a)

The attributes within the inner circle relate to the first psychology and are crucial in helping one to notice and engage with distress and suffering. This begins with care for well-being – a sense of being motivated to care about ourselves and others. Sensitivity relates to our ability to tune into, notice, and engage with suffering, rather than moving away from or avoiding it. Sympathy involves being emotionally moved by one’s own or others’ experiences, but this can bring us into contact with painful feelings, memories, and experiences – and therefore require us to have sufficient tolerance for distress, such that we can manage and regulate contacted experiences. Empathy is an important aspect of compassion, as it allows us to understand and make sense of our own and others' distress and suffering – to see clearly into the nature of it (e.g., its origin, form, triggers, etc.). Although not exhaustive, the final element here is non-judgement: an attempt to not criticise or condone, but rather to *accept* and allow things to be as they are in the moment (even if we may want to bring change to these in the future).

Whilst these above attributes of compassion can be helpful for enabling clients to move towards and engage with distress, in CFT we are also interested in how we might learn to alleviate suffering and prevent it from returning. This is where the second psychology of the outer-circle 'multimodal' skills interventions becomes apparent. These skills can be used to help stimulate some of the inner circle attributes of compassion (motivation, distress tolerance, empathy) which in concert, give rise to a 'compassionate mind' that can be directed to working on the client's difficult experiences in life.

10.4 CFT Interventions

CFT is rooted in the general psychological sciences rather than focusing on a particular process such as cognition, behaviour, or emotion, and then building a therapy around that. CFT focuses on what science tells us about how the evolved brain goes about its tasks; what it needs to function optimally, and what blocks it from doing so. In regard to therapeutic interventions, CFT is highly integrative of other evidence-based interventions such as guided discovery, exposure, imagery, and skills acquisition amongst many others (Gilbert, 2009b; 2010, 2014b).

10.4.1 Attention Training and Mindfulness

As in other approaches, understanding the significant role that attention can have in our distress – and its alleviation – is integral to CFT. What we attend to can have powerful physiological correlates. CFT promotes learning to notice where one's attention tends to lie or get drawn to, and cultivating greater stability of attention on things that are benign or even helpful in alleviating our distress (rather than avoiding it). Attention has overlaps with mindfulness, and in CFT it is important to help clients build their mindfulness skills. When developed, these can be utilised to notice the 'loops in the mind' between new (e.g., typical negative or self-critical thoughts) and old brain (e.g., anxiety or social avoidance), and, rather than remain stuck 'mindlessly' in these, use attention and mindfulness skills to manage these more helpfully.

10.4.2 Soothing Breathing Rhythm

Recent research has suggested that practicing certain types of breathing rhythm, often linked to slowing down and deepening the breath, can have a variety of physiological and psychological benefits (Brown & Gerbarg, 2012), and stimulates parasympathetic/vagal tone (Porges, 2009). There is growing evidence that stimulating the myelinated vagus nerve through various forms of training impacts upon prosocial behaviour (e.g., Kogan et al., 2014). CFT uses these ideas in helping clients to develop a soothing or calming breathing rhythm, in which a sense of grounding and slowing down is practiced.

10.4.3 Imagery

Developing certain types of imagery – particularly those in which affiliative-, care- and compassion-based feelings are evoked – can be important in stimulating emotion (Holmes & Mathews, 2010). CFT focuses on developing imagery to facilitate 'compassion as flow', in which compassion is seen as being experienced in three directions:

(1) From others to self. Here, we help clients to develop and practice an ideal 'compassionate other'. Clients are guided in considering the core qualities and attributes that they would like an ideal compassionate other to have, and, following identification of these, in developing imagery that helps to represent this ideal. Once developed, clients are encouraged and guided to experience compassionate qualities flowing from the image to them.

(2) From self to others. Here, the therapist guides clients, through imagery, acting, and body posture techniques, to help develop their ideal compassionate self. Once this 'self' is developed, clients are encouraged to practice directing this to others: towards people they care for and feel close to, towards strangers, or – when more experienced in this intervention – towards people that they may have more difficult relationships with.

(3) From self to self (self-compassion). Clients are supported to direct compassion-based thoughts and feelings from their 'ideal compassionate self' (developed in [2] above) to themselves. Through self-to-self relating, clients are encouraged to develop a compassionate understanding of the nature of their distress (first circle of compassion), and to facilitate mentalization and courage that may serve to alleviate underlying difficulties.

10.4.4 Directing the 'Compassionate Mind'

Once the ideal compassionate other and ideal compassionate self are developed, CFT therapists will then use a variety of techniques, many of which are derived from other therapeutic approaches, to continue the process of engaging with and alleviating suffering. These include: completion of 'compassionate thought' forms, compassionate letter writing, compassionate chair work, 'multiple self' work, behavioural experiments, and so forth. Some of these are outlined in more detail in Gilbert (2009a).

10.5 CFT: Who Does it Work For and How?

CFT was originally developed as a transdiagnostic approach for people with high levels of shame and self-criticism (Gilbert & Irons, 2005). Leaviss and Uttley (2014) conducted a systematic review of the published literature to date. In a total of 14 studies (including three randomised controlled trials; RCTs) they found initial evidence for effectiveness, particularly in those with high self-criticism. However, they acknowledged that more research is needed before it can be considered to be an evidence-based intervention. Although originally developed to work with transdiagnostic problems like shame and self-criticism, studies have highlighted the potential effectiveness of CFT for people experiencing *psychosis* (e.g., Braehler et al., 2013; Laithwaite et al., 2009), *eating disorders* (e.g., Gale et al., 2014), *personality disorder* (Lucre & Corten, 2013) and *PTSD* (Beaumont, Galpin, & Jenkins, 2012). It is likely therefore that CFT is helpful for presentations that do not manifest with high levels of shame and self-criticism.

There is limited evidence identifying the mechanisms of change in CFT, although early research suggests that the effects of CFT may be mediated via reductions in self-criticism or increases in compassion (e.g., Braehler et al., 2013). It is important to note that, whilst identifying *psychological* mechanisms of change is important for CFT, we are also interested in the underlying *biological* and *physiological* processes involved, for which there already exists a broad scientific evidence-base (e.g., the powerful role of vagal tone and oxytocin on regulating the physiological processes linked to threat and stress; Carter, 2014; Porges, 2009). CFT seeks to build its interventions upon these broader scientific findings. Further large scale trials will be necessary to examine the efficacy of CFT and to develop an understanding of underlying mechanisms of change.

10.6 Criticisms of Compassion Focused Therapy

CFT is a relatively new psychotherapeutic approach, and as such the evidence base is growing but small in comparison to other active, efficacious treatments (e.g., CBT). It is unclear at this stage which components of treatment may be most effective but – as is the case for other process-based approaches (e.g., Dialectical Behavioural Therapy) – it may be difficult to manualise CFT interventions to fit strict RCT criteria. Finally, CFT has been criticised for over-simplifying complex neurophysiological processes (e.g., the heuristic of old brain-new brain, and three affect regulation systems), although these were purposeful simplifications to facilitate practical and experiential understanding in therapists and clients. Moreover, these have been acknowledged in the CFT literature as being just this – i.e., simplifications of highly complex and interacting biological and physiological processes.

10.7 Formulation in Action

There are some key aspects of formulating in CFT:

- Formulations are, where possible, developed *with* clients, in a collaborative manner; with themes 'emerging' in-session, rather than the therapist presenting the client with a formulation that they have worked on between sessions.
- Therapists are encouraged to avoid becoming overly formulaic or restrictive in their method and language of formulating; we are not trying to diagnose or fit people in to boxes that they don't agree with.
- Language used by the therapist is congruent with the theory and principle of de-shaming. CFT therapists do not use terms like 'thinking errors', 'irrational thoughts' or 'maladaptive schema', or try and locate these inside a person, as such problematizing and internalising language can be very shaming for many clients. Rather, it can be more helpful to use normalising and de-shaming language ('it's understandable' and 'not your fault') to enable people to see (1) how their experiences in life have sensitised their threat system, and (2) that many of the behaviours they have engaged in, even if they caused other difficulties, were understandable given the circumstances.
- It can help to build formulations in small steps, particularly for those clients who feel overwhelmed, taking time to help people acclimatise and assimilate (often painful) information about their past experiences and current difficulties.
- Formulation has different functions. For example, to help the clinician and client make sense of what's happening, or for therapeutic planning.
- Two methods of formulating in CFT are: (1) developing a historically based, threat focused formulation, that links historical difficulties to current fears and safety strategies, and (2) a formulation based explicitly around the functioning and 'balance' of a client's 'three systems'. Below, we will highlight aspects of the case material that seemed key to help us formulate using these methods, and identify the links to the theoretical underpinnings of CFT.

10.7.1 Initial Formulations

10.7.1.1 Threat Focused Formulation

The threat focused formulation focuses, as the name suggests, on the nature of threats that Molly struggles with. We are particularly interested in the types of historical experiences that have sensitised the development of her threat system, and the type of key threats that she struggles with in the 'here and now'. We are also concerned about how she has tried to adapt to her environments by developing various safety or protective strategies (either consciously or non-consciously) to manage these threats, and the unintended consequences that have emerged from these strategies. Finally, we attempt to understand how these unintended consequences, via sensitising certain types of (e.g., self-critical) self-to-self relationships, may create a feedback loop (vicious circle) by fuelling current fears and threats.

A diagram of Molly's threat-based, four-column formulation is given in Figure 10.4. Below, we will explore each of the columns in more detail.

Historical influences. The threat focused formulation begins with an exploration of Molly's historical experiences and emotional memories. As noted elsewhere (e.g., Gilbert, 2010), CFT conceptualises emotion in terms of three basic systems, and thus, when assessing historical influences, we are keen to look out for the type of experiences that might have sensitised these, and try to understand how these systems have 'learned', developed, and express themselves.

There appears to be a variety of experiences that might have had a significant impact on Molly. She described experiencing her upbringing as lacking warmth, and it appears that her parents had a distant and emotionally avoidant relationship. It may be that early experiences of her mother being critical of her father behind his back prepared later tendencies to perceive other people as untrustworthy, dishonest, and privately judgmental. Although Molly described feeling very close to and able to rely on her sister, there are also difficulties in this relationship. Molly felt that her sister had an easier life when they were growing up – that she was more loved by their parents, and did not have to work as hard to earn their affection. In comparison, Molly described a sense that, within the family, she was seen as overly emotional, dramatic, and *different* (e.g., being 'ill' and in need of medical care).

Although Molly was liked by her teachers and had some friends, she found it difficult to form and maintain relationships with her peers, and felt that she was 'too controlling' and 'emotionally demanding'. Academically, she was expected to succeed but, from her mother at least, to do this without relying on help from others; moreover, if she failed to achieve as much as expected, she experienced her mother as disappointed in her. As she progressed, successfully, through school and college, she was initially excited about university but increasingly found it difficult to be away from home. Moreover, university posed its own threats; she described feeling 'exposed' in classes, and began avoiding going to classes, assignments, social engagements, and her housemates. After having sex with one of her housemates – during which she experienced significant 'shame', after the other housemates burst in to the room – she felt rejected after trying to get closer to him, and was described as 'clingy'. This was also associated with an increasing sense that people were talking negatively about her – in CFT, this might be an example of *external shame* (Gilbert, 2009b).

Key fears and threats. Variations in our early experiences can create very different mentalities in later life. In a simplistic way, our relational and social experiences can leave us feeling secure, safe, and at ease in relationships and in ourselves; or insecure, threatened, and fearful. There is of course a large literature on how certain types of early experiences are linked to the development of certain fears and threats that carry forward to later life (e.g., Bowlby, 1969; Cassidy & Shaver, 1999), and, as with other therapies, many of these in CFT involve archetypal concerns linked to rejection, abandonment, isolation, shame, and harm (Gilbert, 2010). Key in identifying a person's fears and threats in CFT is to distinguish between external and internal threats.

External threats. External threats relate to concerns that we might have about the outside world (e.g., of harm/attack) and of what other people might think, feel, and do to us (e.g., reject, abandon, criticise). Given her historical experiences discussed above – particularly those linked to relationships with her parents, sister, and friends – it is likely that Molly will be fearful of others rejecting and abandoning her, or of them feeling like she is a burden to them in some way. It is also likely that she will feel concerned with/threatened by others' thinking negatively of her or being critical of her.

Internal threats. Internal threats relate to difficulties that arise inside of us, such as our *emotions* (e.g., becoming overwhelmed by sadness, anxiety, or anger, or even a fear of positive emotions), *feelings* (e.g., vulnerable, alone), *memories*, or more broadly, issues around negative *self-identity* (e.g., self as flawed, bad, defective). Given our knowledge of Molly's experiences in life, and the likely external fears described above, it may be that she struggles with internal feelings of loneliness, weakness, worthlessness, and unloveability. Moreover, we would also hypothesise that she might find the experience and expression of certain emotions – such as anxiety and sadness – quite threatening.

Safety, protective and compensatory strategies. Humans, like other animals, are endowed with a variety of strategies to deal with threats in the world. These are evolved competencies – for example, to seek others for reassurance or to stay away from harm – that can have subtle genetic and temperamental differences, and can also be shaped up through life experiences (Gilbert, 2010). These strategies emerge as ways to regulate threat experiences (threat system) and may differ depending on whether they are aimed at managing an external or internal threat. They often develop in childhood or adolescence, and over time, become reinforced (sometimes through operant conditioning processes; see Chapter 3) and continue to be a feature of adult life. These strategies can again be split between those that attempt to regulate external threats, and those that regulate internal ones.

External safety strategies. To deal with the external threat of rejection by others, it is likely that Molly attempts to seek closeness (e.g., as she did with Danny and Jack), and to appease or please others in some way. In terms of perceiving that others have negative thoughts or perceptions about her, it may be that Molly has developed a heightened sensitivity (vigilance) to monitoring other people (e.g., their reactions to her, or maybe even their facial expression, tone of voice, and moods) to help 'spot' any potential disruptions as early as possible. This may also involve her attempting to employ mindreading (thinking about what others are thinking, based on their reactions and actions towards her). At times, particularly when unable to manage these threats, Molly may try to move away from (avoid) others (as she did during university) to cut off from the threats and fears she experiences around them.

Internal safety strategies. It is likely that, in the face of a number of her internal fears (e.g., feeling unlovable, weak, and worthless) Molly protects herself by suppressing her own needs, distress, and emotions. She might share little with other people and keep much to herself. For many people with similar types of internal fears, self-criticism becomes a safety strategy in that 'it is safer to criticise and blame myself', and the function of this criticism may be to improve herself, or perhaps to punish herself for perceived flaws.

Unintended consequences and self-to-self relating. As with other psychotherapies (e.g., CBT), whilst safety strategies can be effective (at times) in the short-term management of threats and fears, they commonly lead to a variety of undesirable and unintended longer-term consequences. The language of unintended consequences is important here as it reinforces a message of 'not your fault' and can be experienced as de-shaming.

Given the type of *external safety strategies* she might engage in (e.g., trying to please others) it is likely that her needs are often overlooked or missed by friends and family. Moreover, shifting between strategies of approach (e.g., trying to keep people close/pursue close relationships) and avoidance (e.g., avoiding others and socially withdrawing) could leave others finding it difficult to establish consistent relationships with her, ultimately leading her to feel uncared for, abandoned, or rejected. Unfortunately, these feelings re- activate her external protective strategies of withdrawal and avoidance.

Given the internal safety strategies that she might engage in (e.g., suppression, self-criticism), it is likely that she will experience unintended consequences of her needs not being met, a 'bounce back' effect of her emotions building up and bubbling over, and an increased sense of anger at herself and others for the way she feels, and her life situation more generally.

It is worth noting the potential interaction between external threats, strategies, and consequences, and how these may stimulate internal threats, strategies, and unintended consequences. For example, external fears, such as feeling that she is a burden to others, may lead to attempts to avoid and withdraw (safety strategies), with associated unintended consequences of feeling isolated and disconnected. This

Key historical influences (What key historical experiences have influenced Molly?)	**Key fears/threats** (Given historical experiences, what key fears has Molly been left with?)	**Protective/safety strategies** (Given key fears, what safety strategies has Molly developed to protect herself?)	**Unintended consequences** (Have her safety strategies led to any unintended or unforeseen consequences?)
▪ Family life 'lacked warmth' – parents distant from each other, did not communicate with each other; mother was critical behind father's back but did not deal with problems directly ▪ Parents view Molly as overly emotional and dramatic for being tearful ▪ Mother had high academic expectations of her – but expected her to achieve without help from others, and was disappointed if she failed ▪ Sense that her parents loved, favoured, and spoiled her sister more ▪ Physical health problems – only family member to see GP regularly ▪ Sexual abuse ▪ Difficulty forming and maintaining relationships at school ▪ Initially academically successful but struggled when work involved social interaction/communication ▪ Sexual intimacy exposed at University ▪ Partners lose interest, reject, and/or are unfaithful ▪ Sense that others get 'tired' of her, or talk negatively behind her back	**External** Rejection and abandonment Others think negatively/are critical of me Other people are burdened by me **Internal** I am unlovable Feeling alone I am weak I am worthless Expressing certain emotions	**External** Keep people close to me Work out what others think/want (hyper-vigilant for others' reactions to me) Try to please/appease others Avoid/withdraw from others **Internal** Suppress own needs Suppress feelings Criticise self	**External** Others find me overbearing and reject me 'False positives' – misread other's responses Others' take advantage of me Isolated/disconnected **Internal** My needs are not met Emotions 'build up' Feel angry at self and others ↓ **Self-to-self relating** Ruminate and criticise self ↓ **Mood** Decrease in mood

Figure 10.4: Threat focused formulation

type of inner experience (e.g., feeling lonely) is likely to be an internal fear, leading to engagement in safety strategies and unintended consequences. It can be helpful to draw these interactions out with people, and, when moving into the intervention phase of therapy, to clarify the different compassion-based qualities needed to manage these interactions.

Ultimately, we would suggest that these unintended consequences are likely to fuel a particular type of self-to-self relationship, characterised by high levels of self-criticism (Molly intimates these in the assessment, e.g., references to having 'never been enough', being 'weak and useless', and 'not interesting'). These self-critical thoughts, as research has highlighted, may constitute a powerful vulnerability and/or maintaining factor for depression and distress (Blatt, Hart, Quinlan, Leadbeater, & Auerbach, 1993; Teasdale & Cox, 2001). As with other models of psychotherapy (e.g., CBT), the combination of these unintended consequences, self-critical thinking styles, and associated low mood, is likely to create a feedback loop (vicious cycle) to Molly's key fears/threats, 'heating' them up and, consequently, driving the need to engage in safety behaviours which, in turn, further exacerbate unintended consequences.

10.7.1.2 Three System Formulation

The formulation described above is often helpful in bringing together key aspects of past experience, and how these have textured current struggles and attempts to manage. It can help to facilitate wisdom and empathy for one's distress, attempts to cope, and life more generally (an insight in to the nature of one's mind, and the events that have led to distress and difficulties; an understanding that these difficulties are not attributable to personal faults or failings). Another helpful way of formulating in CFT is through the three system (threat, drive, soothing) affect regulation model described earlier in this chapter.

When using a three system formulation, we could ask Molly to focus on the 'here and now' – that is, how she feels each of the three systems functions in her average, day-to-day life (or in an area of life that we know she might struggle in particular with, e.g., relationships). We could also think about the three systems in historical terms, guiding her to consider what experiences from her past sensitised or influenced the development of each system. Below, we will discuss just the 'here and now' understanding.

Current functioning of Molly's 'three systems'. After describing to Molly the basic psychoeducation around the three systems (see above), we would then go on to collaboratively explore each system in turn, focusing on how each currently functions for her. With each system, we would be keen to explore:

Common triggers for activation of this system (including what these are, how often they occur, how long they trigger the system for, whether they are 'external' or 'internal' in origin)

- The type of emotions most common when the system is activated. Here it is key to also explore which emotions may be blocked, avoided, or not experienced (for example, for some people struggling with depression, sadness can be experienced but anger is considered too threatening or dangerous)
- The type of behaviours engaged in when the system is activated (these can also be seen in terms of safety strategies but involve basic evolved defences – e.g., flight, fight, submission, avoidance, etc.)
- The type of thinking styles associated with it. These commonly involve forms of self-criticism, rumination, worry, and a variety of 'better safe than sorry' patterns.
- When thinking about Molly, we could depict her three systems below (in a simplified representation):

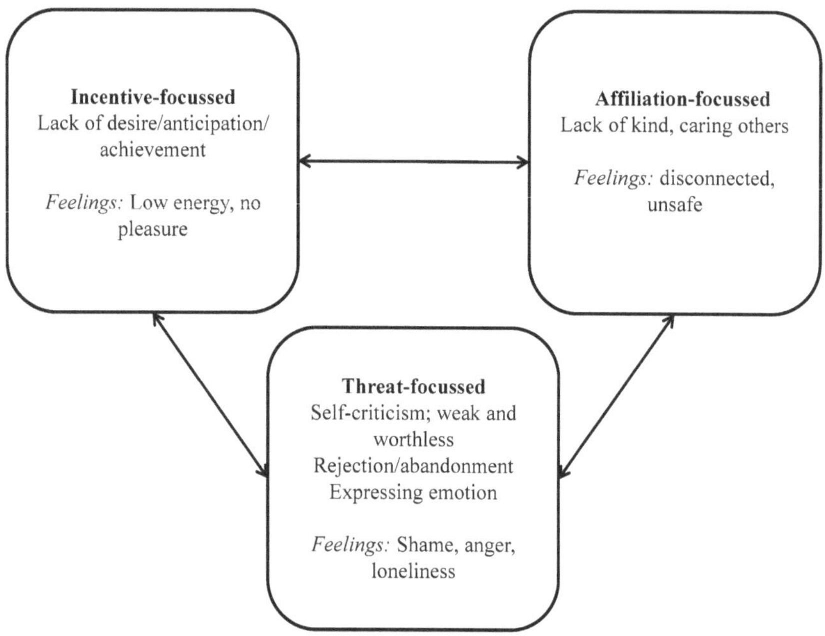

Figure 10.5: Three systems formulation (adapted from Gilbert, 2009a)

Threat system. From a CFT perspective, mental health difficulties and distress often relate to the functioning of the threat system. From a historical point of view, it is clear that Molly had many threat-based experiences during her childhood, adolescence, and young adult life, and we have explored much of this in the threat-based formulation described above. When formulating her current threat system activation, we could help her to consider current external triggers (e.g., sensing that others are critical or burdened by her) and internal triggers (e.g., self-criticism for her problems in life or rumination on events from the past). It is likely that when this system is activated, Molly engages in a variety of defensive behaviours, including avoidance and social withdrawal. She may also struggle to down-regulate certain emotions (shame, anger), and may find the expressing of other emotions and feelings, such as sadness, difficult.

Drive system. The drive system is an important source of motivation, initiative, and energy in moving us towards things that are important in our lives. Unfortunately for Molly, we would hypothesise that she has significant problems in accessing this system in a balanced and consistent way. It is likely that she finds it difficult to feel motivated to pursue things in life (work, a stable boyfriend, friends), partly as this is likely to active her threat system (e.g., concerns about failure, not being good enough, or being abandoned if she did develop a relationship). Moreover, when achievements arrive in life, we would suggest that Molly would find it difficult to experience pleasure from these events. This may partly be due to an over-activation of her threat system, comparing her achievements negatively to others, or a more profound fear of happiness (e.g., Gilbert et al., 2012).

Soothing-affiliative system. The soothing-affiliative system is hypothesised to develop through repeated affectionate and caring experiences through life, and has a powerful impact upon regulating threat system activation. Unsurprisingly, given her historical experiences and developed 'sense of self', we would suggest Molly has significant difficulties accessing her soothing-affiliative system. Given her early experiences (her relationships with her parents and sister, sexual abuse), along with more recent difficulties relating to and developing close relationships with other people, it is likely that she has few external sources of affiliative soothing, reassurance, or contentment. Moreover, if these are actually present, her threat system (linked to shame, rejection, and so forth) is likely to activate in such a way that it down-regulates her capacity to *really* connect with and experience the helpful presence of others. It is likely that she feels disconnected and separate from others, and may find it difficult, at present, to experience family or friends as soothing, calming agents. Moreover, it is likely that Molly will struggle to treat herself with self-reassurance or engage in things for herself that have a soothing/calming function; thus, her internal capacity to stimulate this system is likely to be compromised. Given this, we would expect that she would find it difficult to regulate her own distressing thoughts and feelings, and will therefore be locked in to threat-based protective strategies rather than more helpful, supportive, and encouraging responses and behaviours.

10.7.1.3 Further Information

From the case material provided, there was no information that we felt was superfluous to developing our formulation, although some aspects were more crucial in highlighting key threats and safety strategies, and the development of the different emotion regulation systems.

From a CFT perspective, we would be interested in gaining further information to shape our understanding of Molly. For example, it would be helpful to know about any core emotional memories that may have shaped her sense of self-identity and self-other relationships. We would be keen to learn more about her emotions, and in particular, which negative emotions (e.g., anger, anxiety, sadness, shame, guilt) and positive emotions and feelings (e.g., happiness, joy, contentment) she was able to notice, describe, experience, and express, and which of these she felt blocked to or fearful about. This would help to identify areas for therapeutic work, as developing compassion skills can help clients to move towards, experience, and tolerate the emotions that they find scary and unpleasant. We would also be interested in finding out more about the type of relationship she had with herself (her self-to-self relationship) and, in particular, the nature of her shame and self-criticism.

We would also be interested in further exploring the different responses Molly has when she is threatened. For example, helping her to explore what leads to a more externalising, blaming, or angry response, versus occasions in which she blames or criticises herself. Similarly, it would be helpful to understand more about her attachment style, and how this might help to conceptualise her relationship with others, the way that she relates to herself, and, crucially, the therapeutic relationship.

10.7.2 Intervention Objectives

In the broadest terms, the intervention would involve a mirroring of the definition of compassion as described above: to help Molly become more sensitive to her own suffering, and increase her capacity/ability to find ways of alleviating this suffering. More specifically, within this, we would be keen to:

- Develop – through the formulation(s) – a greater understanding and empathy for the nature of her difficulties and distress, what maintains them (safety strategies), how these lead to a variety of unintended consequences, and how the development of all of these are not her fault, but rather a result of factors that she could not control (e.g., having an evolved brain that is naturally threat sensitive; a set of genes that may predispose difficulties; a variety of early experiences that she did not choose) that left her with high threat activation and low soothing-affiliation.
- Recognise the functioning of her 'three systems' and the effect of imbalance between these systems: the overactive and powerful nature of her threat system, the difficulty in engaging in helpful drive-achievement, and, in particular, the role of the soothing-affiliative system in regulating distress and suffering (either through others or internally through self-compassion).
- Develop the attributes of compassion (inner circle of compassion – Fig. 10.3) to help engage with and facilitate the regulation of affect and her key external and internal threats/fears.

- Develop the skills, strategies, and techniques (outer circle of compassion – Fig. 10.3) to help to alleviate Molly's suffering.

More precisely, we would want to help Molly to develop the above qualities so as to turn towards, and find ways to alleviate, her key fears and threats – as identified in her threat formulation (Fig. 10.4). To help Molly with her fear of rejection and the approach/avoidance protective strategy responses often utilised, we would first help to build capacity in her soothing system (e.g., through breathing and imagery interventions) to enable her to better regulate these fears, before developing specific compassion skills (facilitating courage to tolerate her concerns, and empathy and mentalizing skills to better understand other peoples' thoughts, feelings, and responses/behaviours towards her). We may also seek to reduce her self-criticism – which is likely to be keeping much of her distress and difficulties regarding rejection locked in place – by helping her develop a more compassionate (validating and empathetic) relationship with herself and the difficulties she experiences.

10.7.3 Potential Difficulties Working with Molly

During therapy, we would expect Molly might have a number of difficulties in engagement, motivation to attend sessions, and that, given the description of her initial presentation and previous relationships with others, she may oscillate between a critical-criticised position in relation to the therapist. We would expect that Molly would initially find it very difficult to engage with the concept of 'not your fault', and that she might become quite self-critical and/or angry with this idea and towards the therapist. We would also expect that Molly would find the idea of developing compassion – in particular, the experience of receiving compassion from others and the nurturing of self-compassion – very difficult, and in fact, frightening. Whilst this type of block to or fear of compassion is quite common (Gilbert et al., 2012) it would be important to formulate any difficulties that Molly experiences, and help her to overcome them.

10.7.4 How Would We Measure Progress?

There are multiple ways in which we would want to gauge progress in CFT for Molly. First, we would ask her to complete a number of self-report scales at different stages of therapy. Commonly in CFT, these might include scales that measure *shame and self-criticism* – e.g., the Other as Shamer scale (Goss, Gilbert, & Allan, 1994) or the Forms and Functions of Self-Criticism scale (Gilbert, Clarke, Hempel, Miles, & Irons, 2004) – levels of *self-compassion* (e.g., Self-Compassion Scale; Neff, 2003) and *fears of compassion* (e.g., Fears of Compassion Scale; Gilbert, McEwan, Matos, & Rivis, 2011). We would also look to use a variety of commonly used symptomology measures.

Alongside this, we would also listen for self-reported subjective change, indications that other people in Molly's life had noticed positive changes in her, and of course, our own appraisal of change. Crucially, we would use the initially developed formulation as a guide to progress; in particular, we would look for specific examples and a generalised sense of whether Molly was experiencing a reduction in the key threats, safety strategies, and unintended consequences described in Figure 10.4. Moreover, we would hope to see that when she experiences threats in her life, Molly is able to use the skills acquired in CFT – mindfulness, breathing, imagery, and cognitive/behavioural strategies linked to her 'compassionate mind' – to actively manage experienced threats in different, less deleterious ways. We would also want to see evidence of impact in her everyday life – in terms of her enjoyment at work and development of healthy relationships with work colleagues and friends.

Louise Braham & Sharron Smith

10.8 CFT Formulation: Critical Commentary

We could firstly identify a number of similarities between our Integrative approach and the approach of Compassion Focused Therapy (CFT). These include having a strong basis in cognitive-behavioural theorising, alongside acknowledging the importance of supportive relationships in facilitating learning of healthier emotion-regulation strategies. The CFT approach certainly has something to offer our understanding of how to engage someone therapeutically, the importance of holding in mind the human condition, and our need for compassion. CFT integrates many of the same literatures that our Assimilative integration did, and the approach is theoretically based in a number of stories that might enable clients to feel that their difficulties are 'not their fault', whilst simultaneously opening up possibilities for change. CFT was developed in response to clinical need, and the rationale for its approach to treatment seems intuitively sensible when thinking about clients in distress and our responses to them. The mismatch described between changed cognitions and unchanged emotions offers an example of how a lack of personal integration could be associated with poor mental health.

However, in considering criticisms of the CFT approach outlined here, it seems that the model might be characterised as overly constrained by its focus on evolutionary accounts of development and the 'all healing' nature of compassion, but also appears to lack theoretical specificity in some areas. For example, what is the mechanism by which self-to-self compassion occurs? How does one become compassionate to oneself? Is a lack of self-compassion at the root of all difficulties or just some of them? If it is just some difficulties, which ones, and how can we tell?

Additionally, CFT promotes an evolutionary account of brain development that might not fit with clients' other beliefs; particularly, perhaps, religious belief systems.

It was not clear to us if this would suggest the approach was inappropriate for religious clients or if there is any adjustment that might enable therapists to minimise this aspect of the work, and hence its potential conflict with the client's broader beliefs. Are there other clients who are unsuitable candidates for CFT intervention?

Further, the authors suggest that CFT interventions are developed on the basis of broader scientific findings relating to physiological processes underpinning stress. Cognitive, behavioural, and neuropsychological models already do this adequately and many such models are well-developed. Given this, does CFT offer anything distinct to our understanding of psychological distress other than the idea that compassion might be a focus for intervention?

How an individual relates to others in the world, and within their mind, is central to their experiences and, consequently, is often implicated in their distress. However, these (external and internal) relationships are poorly explicated within this account of a CFT approach. The account does not sufficiently explain how Molly relates to others, or how her relational style and others' expectations of her might impact on her relationship difficulties. At the level of formulation, we wondered about the advantages and disadvantages of using a 'threat based' or 'three systems' approach to formulating; how the information gathered by these formulations would inform the treatment approach; and how to choose between these approaches at different points in therapy.

Essentially, the authors seemed likely to choose between a very limited range of specific treatment-approaches, on the basis of supportive efficacy research and clinical judgement. Although this mirrored our Assimilative integration approach, CFT appeared more constrained in terms of the treatment approaches it draws upon, due to an over-focus on compassion-development – despite the lack of clear evidence to suggest that this construct is more important or central than others when working with clients.

There is an acknowledged emphasis on distinguishing internal and external factors in understanding safety behaviours, but this separation might contribute to a limited conceptualisation of how these factors may interact. By trying to conceptualise the separation of internal and external factors, we would be concerned that important information is needlessly neglected within the formulation.

We are aware that, to date, there is limited evidence regarding CFT outcomes – and, of course, psychological therapies are continually developing in terms of their evidence-base. Perhaps we could consider CFT as being in its infancy as a theory and treatment approach, with a number of large steps yet to be taken. As an integrative approach, it is a challenge to know the extent to which you need to specify the bases of your theoretical allegiances and how to do this concisely enough to cover the material within a single chapter. Any explanation can only ever be partial and limited, and we value accounts that simplify complex processes as useful explanatory guides for clients. CFT offers a framework for a particular way of understanding patterns of relationships and distress that some clients may find useful. However, we would question the assumptive focus on compassion, shame, and self-criticism as central factors (underlying difficulties) for all clients, particularly when the thinking around these concepts and inter-relationships remains inchoate.

Vanessa Dale-Hewitt & Chris Irons

10.9 Author response

There are a number of points raised by the commentators that we do not feel accurately reflect CFT as an approach.

First, it is unclear how an approach can be 'overly constrained' by an evolutionary understanding of the human mind, distress, and mental healthiness – evolutionary understanding underpins many psychotherapeutic approaches, and provides a basic scientific grounding for clients and therapists. Of course, for some clients an evolutionary explanation may not fit with their broader beliefs, but, in our experience, key aspects of the approach (e.g., old/new brain, three systems) still stand as helpful psychoeducational heuristics even without an evolutionary back story.

Second, whilst compassion may not be a panacea, there is a large and rapidly developing scientific literature – both from within psychotherapy research and more broadly – that highlights how the cultivation of compassion for self and others, and the experience of receiving compassion, is highly physiologically and psychologically regulating for humans. There is emerging evidence of how compassion may be associated with epigenetic changes, immunological improvements, improvements in heart-rate variability, reduction in negative affect and mental health symptomology, satisfaction in relationships, and altruism. These are not studies that CFT has directed, but certainly we are interested in what the scientific literature is telling us about the consequences of cultivating compassion. We would also like to highlight that, whilst cultivating the different flows of compassion is central to the approach, CFT embraces and uses a variety of other interventions (e.g., attention training, mindfulness) that fit coherently within the model and are likely to be important components of therapeutic change.

Third, whilst we clearly highlighted that CFT emerged initially through working with people who had high levels of shame and self-criticism, the approach is also used with people who do not have problems in these areas. Given much of mental health distress involves high threat processing, the CFT model, with its focus on threat regulation, has much to offer.

Fourth, in regard to the scientific understanding of the physiology of stress, we are unclear about the commentators' point that "cognitive, behavioural and neuropsychological models already do this adequately and many models are very well developed". It is unclear which of these models try to base their theoretical understanding or interventions on a similar underlying physiological model – incorporating an understanding of polyvagal theory (Porges, 2007) or the powerful role of oxytocin in regulating stress systems. We do not agree that CFT is "in its infancy as a theory and treatment approach" – in fact we would suggest that there is a great deal of depth and integration across multiple levels of psychological and biological science – but certainly expect adaptations and developments in years to come.

In terms of formulation itself, of course there is a lot in the process that is hard to convey here. Contrary to the commentators' concerns, we find that failure to explicitly separate external and internal processes can lead to confusion. But of course it is important to recognise how external and internal processes interact, and drawing out these interactions is a key process in CFT formulation and understanding.

References

Beaumont, E. A., Galpin, A. J., & Jenkins, P. E. (2012). 'Being kinder to myself': A prospective comparative study, exploring posttrauma therapy outcome measures, for two groups of clients, receiving either cognitive behaviour therapy or cognitive behaviour therapy and compassionate mind training. *Counselling Psychology Review, 27*(1), 31-43.

Belsky, J., & Pluess, M. (2009). Beyond diathesis stress: differential susceptibility to environmental influences. *Psychological Bulletin, 135*(6), 885.

Blatt, S. J., Hart, B., Quinlan, D. M., Leadbeater, B., & Auerbach, J. (1993). Interpersonal and self-critical dysphoria and behavioral problems in adolescents. *Journal of Youth and Adolescence, 22*(3), 253-269.

Bowlby, J. (1969). *Attachment and loss: Vol. 1. Attachment.* London: Penguin.

Braehler, C., Gumley, A., Harper, J., Wallace, S., Norrie, J., & Gilbert, P. (2013). Exploring change processes in compassion focused therapy in psychosis: Results of a feasibility randomized controlled trial. *British Journal of Clinical Psychology, 52*(2), 199-214.

Brown, R., & Gerbarg, P. (2012). *The healing power of the breath: Simple techniques to reduce stress and anxiety, enhance concentration, and balance your emotions.* Boston, MA: Shambhala Publications.

Carter, C. S. (2014). Oxytocin pathways and the evolution of human behavior. *Annual Review of Psychology, 65*, 17-39.

Cassidy, J., & Shaver, P. R. (1999). *Handbook of attachment: Theory, research, and clinical applications.* New York: Guilford Press.

Cozolino, L. (2007). *The neuroscience of human relationships: Attachment and the developing brain.* New York: Norton.

Depue, R. A., & Morrone-Strupinsky, J. V. (2005). A neurobehavioral model of affiliative bonding: Implications for conceptualizing a human trait of affiliation. *Behavioral and Brain Sciences, 28*(3), 313-349.

Gale, C., Gilbert, P., Read, N., & Goss, K. (2014). An evaluation of the impact of introducing compassion focused therapy to a standard treatment programme for people with eating disorders. *Clinical Psychology & Psychotherapy, 21*(1), 1-12.

Gilbert, P. (2009a). *The compassionate mind.* London: Constable & Robinson.

Gilbert, P. (2009b). Introducing compassion-focused therapy. *Advances in Psychiatric Treatment, 15*(3), 199-208.

Gilbert, P. (2010). *Compassion focused therapy: Distinctive features.* London: Routledge.

Gilbert, P. (2014). Compassion-focused therapy: Preface and introduction for special section. *British Journal of Clinical Psychology, 53*(1), 1-5.

Gilbert, P., Clarke, M., Hempel, S., Miles, J., & Irons, C. (2004). Criticizing and reassuring oneself: An exploration of forms, styles and reasons in female students. *British Journal of Clinical Psychology, 43*(1), 31-50.

Gilbert, P., & Choden. (2013). *Mindful Compassion: Using the power of mindfulness and compassion to transform our lives*. London: Constable & Robinson Ltd.

Gilbert, P., & Irons, C. (2005). Focused therapies and compassionate mind training for shame and self-attacking. In P. Gilbert (Ed.), *Compassion: Conceptualisations, research and use in psychotherapy* (pp. 263-325). London: Routledge.

Gilbert, P., McEwan, K., Gibbons, L., Chotai, S., Duarte, J., & Matos, M. (2012). Fears of compassion and happiness in relation to alexithymia, mindfulness, and self-criticism. *Psychology and Psychotherapy: Theory, Research and Practice, 85*(4), 374-390.

Gilbert, P., McEwan, K., Matos, M., & Rivis, A. (2011). Fears of compassion: Development of three self-report measures. *Psychology and Psychotherapy: Theory, Research and Practice, 84*(3), 239-255.

Goss, K., Gilbert, P., & Allan, S. (1994). An exploration of shame measures—I: The other as shamer scale. *Personality and Individual Differences, 17*(5), 713-717.

Holmes, E. A., & Mathews, A. (2010). Mental imagery in emotion and emotional disorders. *Clinical Psychology Review, 30*(3), 349-362.

Kogan, A., Oveis, C., Carr, E., Gruber, J., Mauss, I., Shallcross, A., . . . Cheng, C. (2014). Vagal activity is quadratically related to prosocial traits, prosocial emotions, and observer perceptions of prosociality. *Journal of Personality and Social Psychology, 107*(6), 1051-1063.

Laithwaite, H., O'Hanlon, M., Collins, P., Doyle, P., Abraham, L., Porter, S., & Gumley, A. (2009). Recovery after psychosis (RAP): A compassion focused programme for individuals residing in high security settings. *Behavioural and Cognitive Psychotherapy, 37*(5), 511-526.

Leaviss, J., & Uttley, L. (2014). Psychotherapeutic benefits of compassion-focused therapy: an early systematic review. *Psychological Medicine, FirstView*, 1-19. doi: doi:10.1017/S0033291714002141

Masterpasqua, F. (2009). Psychology and epigenetics. *Review of General Psychology, 13*(3), 194-201.

Neff, K. D. (2003). The development and validation of a scale to measure self-compassion. *Self and Identity, 2*(3), 223-250.

Panksepp, J. (1998). *Affective neuroscience: The foundations of human and animal emotions*. New York: Oxford University Press.

Porges, S. W. (2009). The polyvagal theory: New insights into adaptive reactions of the autonomic nervous system. *Cleveland Clinic Journal of Medicine, 76*(Suppl 2), S86-S90. doi: 10.3949/ccjm.76.s2.17

Stott, R. (2007). When head and heart do not agree: A theoretical and clinical analysis of rational-emotional dissociation (RED) in cognitive therapy. *Journal of Cognitive Psychotherapy, 21*(1), 37-50.

Teasdale, J. D., & Cox, S. G. (2001). Dysphoria: self-devaluative and affective components in recovered depressed patients and never depressed controls. *Psychological Medicine, 31*(07), 1311-1316.

Westbrook, D., Kennerley, H., & Kirk, J. (2011). *An introduction to Cognitive Behaviour Therapy: Skills and applications*. London: Sage.

Louise Braham, Danielle De Boos & Sharron Smith

11 Integrative Approaches

Integration might be more appropriately seen as a movement than an approach; a movement that has involved the development of myriad ways of 'doing' integration. Integrative working has been borne from the explosive proliferation of, and resulting heterogeneity in, psychotherapy approaches, and it is clear to us that there is little value in attempting to convey any myth of uniformity in this chapter. To suggest that there is a single integrative approach that can be learnt and followed would be misleading: integrative working draws on the full range of possible theories about human distress and psychological routes to change and wellbeing, and therefore the possible combinations and permutations within integrative working are limitless.

Integrative working has evolved under a range of favourable conditions. Without doubt, one such condition has been an increasingly widespread recognition that no single theoretical model or approach to psychotherapy has all of the answers, for all of the people, all of the time. This, alongside a drive to constantly improve the efficiency, efficacy, and acceptability of psychotherapy, has led clinicians, academics, and researchers alike to look across the range of psychotherapy approaches in order to refine, elaborate, and improve the way we work. To that end, integrative working aims to be flexible and responsive to the needs and competence of both client and therapist, with the goal of improving outcomes.

In this chapter, we have been asked to consider what is unique about integrative working. This is a tricky question to answer. In one sense, nothing is unique about integrative working because it rests entirely on the foundations built by 'pure-form' models and approaches: the process of integrating individual approaches is (and we argue, should be) based on the evidence-base for each approach being drawn upon. We appreciate a specific point of wisdom from John Norcross in his book on the subject (2005) that "one cannot integrate what one does not know" (p.14). We note also that the approaches considered in other chapters of this text are, in many cases, works of integration themselves. Our sense is that perhaps what is unique about integrative working is the opportunity to refrain from repeatedly redefining and 're-badging' through the demarcation of new boundaries; rather, integrative working might be seen as a 'meta-approach' in which all approaches are held in mind and applied dynamically. More generally though, we wish to communicate that integrative working is a natural extension and evolution of pure-form working, rather than a theoretical opponent to it.

11.1 The Origins of Integrative Working

The origins of integrative working offer much by way of explanation of its philosophy. In the 1950s and 1960s key psychotherapeutic 'camps' (psychoanalysis, behaviourism, cognitivism) were engaged competitively with each other to prove the value of their respective approaches. This is described by some authors as akin to an 'ideological cold war' (Norcross, 2005) and the difficulty we have today in imagining this level of furious duelling is perhaps testament to the impact that the integrative movement has had in the last forty years. Ultimately, they were all shown to be effective for some people and the differences between them were judged to be small and unreliable (Wampold, 2001; Wampold et al., 1997). The resulting 'all have won and all shall have prizes' conclusion (the 'Dodo verdict'; Rosenzweig, 1936), when combined with findings that a larger portion of change could be attributed to client variables and common factors than to the specific model itself, led to something of a revolution.

The first identifiably integrative publication came in 1950 (Dollard & Miller, Personality and Psychotherapy) but it took until the 1970s for the movement towards integrative working to gather any significant pace (Prochaska, 1979; Wachtel, 1977). The conditions were right for integration, not simply by virtue of outcome-related dissatisfaction with any single-model approach; short-term approaches to psychotherapy became more numerous and credible, and alongside this the financial and organisational support for traditional long-term approaches began to dwindle. Therapists were asked anew to demonstrate and document the efficacy of their approach, leading to a favouring of more easily-evidenced, problem-focussed ways of working with clients. There was an additional sense of theoretical dissatisfaction that no single theory could fully explain or predict the development of core concepts like personality, or the aetiology of clinical problems and why they change. Academics began peering over the fences to see what neighbouring theories could offer and a timely increase in collaboration between academics and clinicians saw this translate into the approaches used in clinical services. Ultimately the movement gathered enough momentum to see the launch of the first journal dedicated to the integrative cause (The International Journal of Eclectic Psychotherapy) in 1982, and professional bodies committed to furthering integrative working followed.

As it stands today, it seems fair to say that a significant move towards integrative working has taken place and is continuing (Prochaska & Norcross, 2010) to the point that most practitioners would identify themselves as either explicitly integrative or at least influenced by more than one theoretical approach (McLeod, 2009). This prompts us to question what the logical end point of this movement might be: Will we arrive at theoretical unification, whereby an ultimate integration of theory and approach is agreed upon as the most effective or universally applicable? We find this almost as difficult to imagine as the 'cold war' described by Norcross. Our sense is that we may instead be experiencing a new proliferation of standardised integrative approaches, for example: Cognitive Behavioural Therapy; Cognitive Analytic Therapy (Ryle, 1995); and Schema therapy (Young, Klosko, & Weishaar, 2003) to name just a few.

11.2 Approaches to Integrative Working

Different forms of integrative working have been defined as ways of classifying approaches. These are briefly discussed to provide context for the approach we intend to take. One factor upon which these ways of integrating vary is the level at which integration occurs: technique, theory, or somewhere between the two.

At the level of *technique*, 'technical eclecticism' involves the collation of therapy techniques that 'work' without necessarily blending the theoretical assumptions underpinning those techniques. An eclectic therapist would not be held to one set of assumptions about how clinical problems operate and they may be less concerned with 'why' something works than the fact that it does work. Technical eclecticism is criticised for inconsistency and potential theoretical muddlement. However Norcross (2005) argues that successful technical eclecticism should involve the systematic selection of techniques on the basis of both outcome research and patient need. Furthermore, to do this he suggests a sound knowledge and experience of several therapeutic approaches is needed.

At the level of *practice*, 'assimilative integration' might be seen as a step towards integration of theory, whilst remaining essentially at the level of practice. This approach begins with a grounding in one 'home' theoretical position and works towards selectively incorporating practices and views from other theories in a process of reworking, augmenting, and casting in new form the ideas from the home theory. Without the demand for full theoretical synthesis, a perspective on theoretical congruence can be adopted. It might be thought of as the way in which therapists naturally expand their clinical repertoire upon recognising the limitations of their home theory.

At the level of *theory*, 'theoretical integration' aims to synthesise different theories that may hold differing world views and underpinning assumptions. Such synthesis offers the potential for new perspectives at a theory level, although the barriers to synthesis should not be underestimated; how do we rationalise assumptions that appear to sit at odds with each other and fundamental epistemological contrasts? A simple example might be the challenge of identifying the aim of therapy; differing theories would support differing objectives, with possible focal outcomes including: the promotion of self-actualisation, the relief of symptoms, the restructuring of relationships, the development of insight, and the modification of overt behaviours. Theoretical integration might seem therefore to present the greatest challenge to a therapist working integratively.

In our view at least, the 'common factors' approach to psychotherapy integration is located somewhere to the side of the 'technique – theory' continuum described above. It has developed from the search for the key ingredients that different therapies share, given the acknowledgment that theoretical nuances do not produce significant variance in efficacy. The process of identifying these common factors has, more recently, included empirical (as well as rational) methods (Grencavage & Norcross, 1990; Tracey, Lichtenberg, Goodyear, Claiborn, & Wampold, 2003). Factors shared across successful therapies are thought to include concepts like alliance; empathy; positive regard; client feedback and preferences; and acknowledgement of culture (Norcross, 2011). Whilst identifying the ingredients of good therapy is undoubtedly valuable, it does not offer an approach for case formulation. We see the common factors approach as a meta-approach: a clinical strategy or arrangement of ideas that guides the efforts of therapists. It does not dictate how theory is to be arranged within that structure and this falls, as it does with other integrative approaches, to the individual therapist to negotiate according to their own preferences, experiences, and resources.

Perhaps in response to this, some 'framework' approaches have offered conceptual maps that organise elements of a clinical case and link these to appropriate theoretical approaches. Jeff Brook-Harris' (2008) Multitheoretical psychotherapy (MTP) approach suggests that 'thoughts', 'actions', and 'feelings', as primary dimensions of human functioning, are influenced by contextual dimensions of 'biology', 'interpersonal patterns', 'social systems', and 'cultural contexts'. MTP goes on to suggest that multiple theories should be considered: e.g., cognitive theory for 'thoughts'; experiential theory for feelings; psychodynamic theory for interpersonal patterns; and so forth. This clearly moves towards an approach for case formulation and the same may be said for other frameworks (Ingram, 2006; Weerasekera, 1996). Ingram's work in particular offers a highly prescriptive approach to the building of a case formulation from individual hypotheses situated within a range of theoretical perspectives. Our sense is that, whilst these frameworks acknowledge the need for some level of theoretical integration, they give little sense of how this might be done.

Our aim in this chapter is to offer an example of the approach we feel most closely represents 'normal integrative practice' for clinicians: assimilative integration. The process we went through to arrive at and execute this is described in more detail in the 'Formulation in Action' section below. Central to our rationale for this decision are two considerations: firstly, what merit is there in reorganising (already frequently reorganised) concepts to produce another framework approach? Secondly, the significant challenges to full theoretical integration mean that this does not reflect real-life practice as we know it. We settled on the notion that producing something with clear relevance for practice was a more pragmatic and useful endeavour.

11.3 What Evidence is There for Integrative Working?

We hope to have ultimately made clear that uniformity within integrative working is indeed a myth. Working integratively can be approached in a number of ways, each of which comes with inherent strengths and limitations.

The evidence-base for integrative working therefore mirrors this lack of uniformity. The evidence specific to each 'branded' theoretically integrated model (e.g., Schema Therapy, Cognitive Analytic Therapy, Cognitive-Behavioural Therapy, and Compassion Focused Therapy) is variously developed and a fuller account of three such models (Schema Therapy, Compassion-Focused Therapy, and Cognitive-Behavioural Therapy) can be seen in previous chapters. Other approaches to working integratively depend on the evidence-base of each model being drawn upon and this extends to the evidence for specific techniques that may exist. In a sense, therefore, many ways of working integratively are difficult to test, given that each is developed in response to a specific problem, for a specific client, by a specific therapist. This affords opportunity for sweeping criticisms of integrative working: that it is untestable and therefore unsound, or lacking in depth, clarity, coherence, and focus (Gilbert & Orlans, 2011).

These criticisms are entirely appropriate when levelled at poor quality integrative working – i.e., unsystematic, 'pick-n-mix' therapy that gives little consideration to congruence, efficacy, or competence. We would argue therefore that integrative working must involve the following:

A thorough and detailed understanding of each theoretical model that is being drawn upon, its evidence-base, and translation to clinical practice.

- Consideration of the idea of theoretical congruence so that the overall message communicated to the client, by the therapy, is coherent.
- As clear a focus on the clinical problem as would be taken by a single-model approach.
- A clear sense, for each therapist, of their own fields of competence and an acceptance that only what is fully understood should be used.

11.4 Formulation in Action

Originally, in thinking about Molly we attempted to develop a novel conceptual model of case formulation, rather like a 'framework' approach. However, it became apparent that this is not how we work with real clients; therefore, we should do as we would in actual practice. This shift allowed us to lose the constraints of trying to produce an all-encompassing, yet clinically usable model of functioning, and indeed also of the challenge of synthesising theory to the point of providing new perspectives. Instead we could work intuitively, starting from a Cognitive-Behavioural Therapy

(CBT) outline. This matched our clinical expertise and was congruent with Molly's tendency to prominently articulate her thoughts and feelings.

The process of assimilative integration allowed us to take note of, and respond to, 'gaps' left by the CBT model. We felt that there were significant systemic and relational aspects to her experience; hence, we augmented our initial CBT formulation with ideas from systemic and psychodynamic approaches. At each stage we considered the theoretical congruence to ensure that the ideas we were using could sit sensibly alongside each other. For the sake of clarity, we will demonstrate our formulation in three stages.

11.4.1 Initial Formulation

11.4.1.1 Stage 1: CBT Model

Figure 11.1 shows application of a Beckian longitudinal CBT model. This model explains the influence of life experiences via the development of core beliefs and rules for living, which are activated and/or violated by more recent trigger events. The model captures Molly's articulation of her self-concept (as 'weak and useless') and is helpful in identifying the connections between longstanding ways of coping and current patterns of thinking, feeling, and behaving. Molly wishes to 'sort (herself) out' and locates her problems internally, which is congruent with CBT assumptions about internal processes driving distress. Please refer to Figure 11.1.

This model is not as useful when it comes to explaining the influence of her family interactions on her current distress, or indeed why, in new situations, she finds similar forms of emotional distress.

11.4.1.2 Stage 2: Addition of Systemic Ideas

As Chapter 8 explains, systemic approaches are informed by systems theory and the notion that the behaviour of a system can be understood by considering the characteristics of each element within the system and the relationship between these elements. Although there is limited information about the wider culture that influences Molly, a system of primary importance in her life is family; there may therefore be value in conceptualising how Molly and her family communicate with each other and the interpersonal aspects of her distress.

Molly's account suggests that her family may have been invested in a system of beliefs around the importance of achievement and of self-reliance (that she should be able to achieve without relying on help from others) and these beliefs seem to have been communicated within the family system through both the language used and in non-verbal communications (her Mother's 'looks'). The family system also seems to favour the non-expression of emotion as part of its overall pattern of communication. As a part of the family system, Molly is likely to have been influenced to maintain these values in her own patterns of communication and behaviour, perhaps to the point that she ‘owns’ them as her own values. She attempts to contain her emotions (‘you just have to get on with it’) but struggles to sustain this and is inevitably overwhelmed, leading to an intensified expression of emotional distress, which the system receives with difficulty.

Interactional patterns within the family system appear to discourage and even punish emotional expression, and this can be observed in the family’s response to Molly’s hospitalisation and in their descriptions of Molly as “overly emotional” and “dramatic”. It is plausible that the family are invested in a wider social discourse about mental health problems reflecting weakness (Molly certainly perceives that they felt stigmatised by having a daughter “in the nuthouse”) as congruent with their own belief system about self-reliance/resilience. This might complement a strategic perspective in proposing that the family’s responses to her distress are, in fact, attempts to encourage resilience in Molly. However, she reports distress resulting from these interactions, which suggests they are ineffective solutions that require disruption.

Molly describes a lack of warmth and an atmosphere of ‘separateness’ within the family system. It may be that when combined with a pattern of communication that discourages expression of emotional distress, this maintains a sense that the system would not receive well any news of traumatic events. Molly chose not to disclose the sexual abuse she suffered, perhaps fearing her account would be understood through the existing family story, in which she is “dramatic” and disclosure would “wreck the family”. This supports the notion that she strived to maintain stability within the system, even though her own need for support was unmet.

Molly has tried to achieve self-reliance, autonomy, and success in a series of transitions (leaving home for university, commencing a relationship, taking a job at the library) that see her joining new systems. Unfortunately this seems to have brought her into contact with some overwhelmingly challenging interactions that have resulted ultimately in a retreat from autonomy (leaving the family system undisrupted). Her distress within these new systems seems to arise from an interaction between her own expectations (that she would be exposed and would fail at university; that she may be rejected in relationships) and the system’s expectations and responses to her behaviour. We hypothesise that a university class culture that expects members to join in and work together may not respond well to increased withdrawal; likewise, a student culture with expectations of casual relationships may not receive well intense attachment behaviours. Hence, Molly finds herself failing to meet others’ expectations, ‘rejected’, and needing to retreat to a position of relative safety. The sense overall is one of repeating patterns within new systems, and the advantage of a systemic understanding is that it facilitates causation and maintenance to be viewed as circular, rather than linear, and solely internally located in Molly.

The augmentation of the CBT formulation with systemic ideas contributes an interpersonal and interactional understanding of Molly’s experience of distress. The CBT formulation acknowledges her tendency to be self-critical of her distress and we feel that a balance needs to be struck between identifying internally-held beliefs and expectations, and recognising the influence of others around her. This offers an alternative perspective on the causation and maintenance of Molly's distress, and in therapy will give us an effective way of dealing with the idea that she is the sole source of her own distress. It is important to state (although this should be obvious) that systemic thinking does not simply transfer responsibility for Molly's distress to people around her; rather, it suggests that systems respond in order to try and achieve stability, purpose, or indeed to solve problems. Molly's distress is understood as arising from these interactions.

11.4.1.3 Stage 3: Addition of Relational Psychodynamic Ideas

The final stage of formulation considers how a relational psychodynamic perspective can add to our understanding of how the systems that Molly grew up in can become internalised and influence her responses to others in the present. Whilst the field of psychodynamic theories is more complex and multifaceted than we have space to explore here, drawing on some essential concepts can usefully add to our developing understanding of Molly. Whereas CBT and systemic approaches tend to address aspects of Molly's experience that she is at least somewhat conscious of, psychodynamic theorising highlights the role of her unconscious in shaping the experience and expression of her difficulties.

Attachment theory and research (Bowlby, 1969, 1973) suggest that a mother's empathic responding to her infant is crucial to the child's development. A caregiver's attunement to their child's experience is regarded as enabling the infant to integrate and organise their experience, later supporting the development of memory, emotion regulation abilities, and a sense of self (Stern, 1985). Given the discouragement of emotional expression within Molly's family, it is likely that her early development was lacking in this vital emotional responsiveness, with consequent effects upon her implicit abilities and her Internal Working Models (IWM; Bowlby, 1969, 1973) of relating to others. Whilst a CBT perspective highlights Molly's 'core beliefs', the IWM concept offers a similar but more dynamic interpersonal understanding of Molly's expectations in relationships, and ways of being with others and the world. The advantage of including a psychodynamic perspective is to support a clearer understanding of how she might shift and change in her thoughts, feelings, and behaviours with others.

Consider, for example, Molly's behaviour in her first therapeutic session: fluctuating between angry criticism of the therapist and apologetic frustration with herself. Such behaviour can be understood as mirroring the conflict experienced by an infant whose mother is unresponsive to their needs. The unmet need creates a sense of angry frustration in the child that they struggle to manage without support, but to survive they still require proximity, and whatever support and safety their caregiver can offer. Consequently, the child is understood to become rejecting of their own needs in order

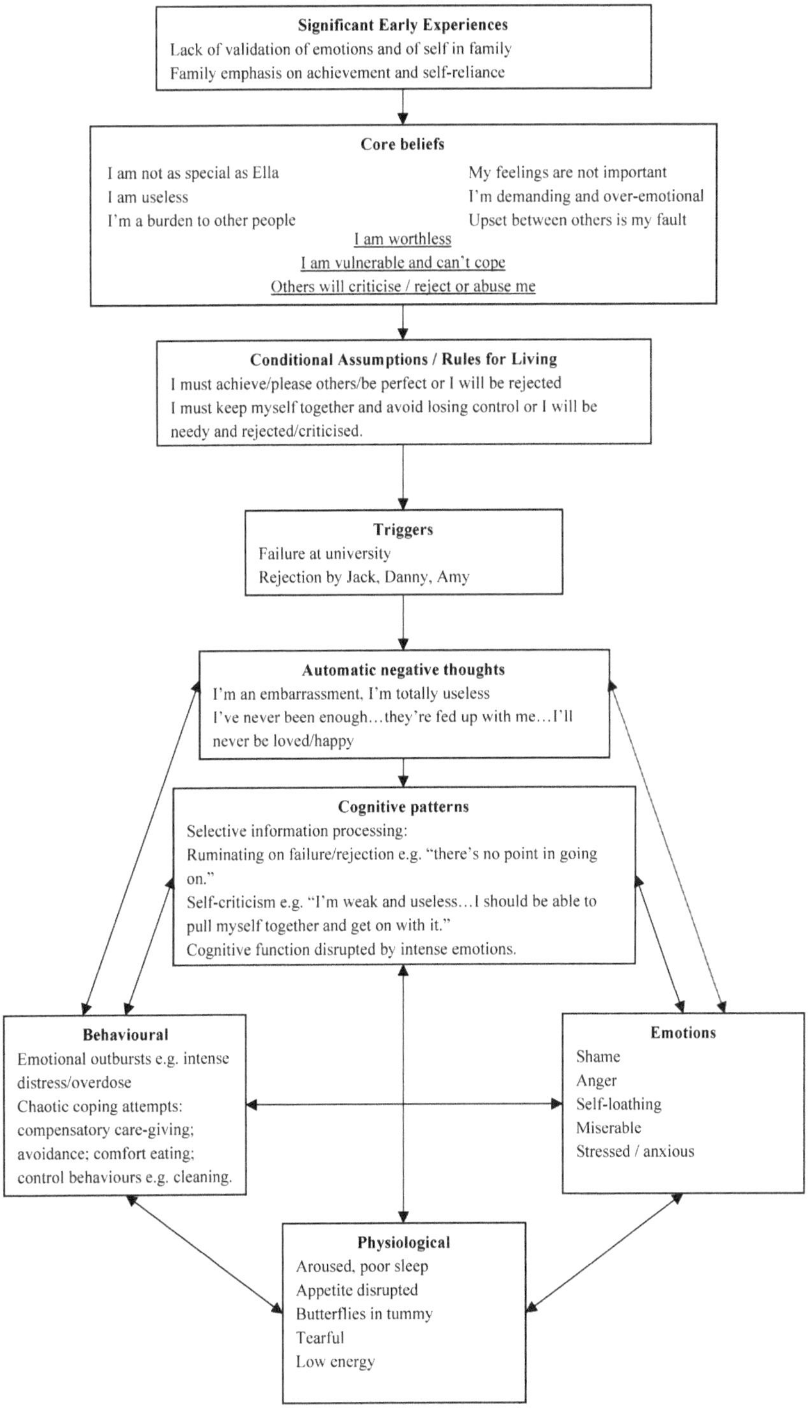

Figure 11.1: CBT diagrammatic formulation

to limit frustration with the caregiver and maintain a compromised relationship. Returning to Molly in the session, we can see this conflict between frustrated needs for emotional support being expressed in her anger, but to guard against the therapist rejecting her, she resorts to criticising herself for not being able to contain the feeling. Unconsciously, Molly's IWM of others as failing to provide for her 'excessive' emotional needs is reconfirmed.

From a relational psychodynamic perspective, Molly could be seen as consciously seeking change, but unconsciously she might feel threatened by insights that undermine her IWMs because they have helped her to maintain a degree of security. Molly may defend against the threat of change in many ways that she could gain insight into, but the risk of her rejecting the therapy and/or therapy relationship is one potential defence that seems crucial to attend to.

We note that the tasks of therapy, such as self-reflection and emotional expression, will be at odds with Molly's usual ways of being in the world. Consequently, maintaining sensitive awareness of Molly's experience of the therapy could provide an opportunity to learn about her relational difficulties, as well as help to guard against a premature ending to the work. The simplified but main tenets of these and the systemic ideas are highlighted in Figure 11.2.

11.4.2 Theoretical Congruence

We have advocated the importance of considering the congruence of the underpinning theories that an integrative formulation may draw upon. This is driven primarily by the need to create a coherent sense of the therapy experience for the client. One area for consideration is the extent to which our models understand 'problems' to be internally or externally located, because this poses a potential conflict of basic assumptions. Our understanding is that Molly's difficulties exist both internally and externally; in fact, to suggest that a raft of life struggles such as those Molly presents with, might have a single location or source, seems unfeasibly simplistic. Put simplistically, CBT understands problems as arising from maladaptive internal processes, whilst systemic theory would identify problems as arising within interactions or relationships. The psychodynamic concept of an IWM offers us a way of bridging this potential divide; suggesting that perhaps the interactions within a family system are formative of an IWM, which comprises internalised processes like emotional regulation and beliefs about the self. Essentially, the ideas and interactions of her family system become Molly's own ideas about herself and the world. Thus her difficulties 'exist' in her interactions with systems, and within her own conscious and unconscious internal experience.

The CBT model offers Molly a way of gaining a sense of conscious control, and therefore hopefully choice, over her experience. It offers a way of capturing and conceptualising her current talk about herself (as core beliefs or rules for living) and the therapy techniques that spring from the model will offer practical challenges to that talk and tools with which to manage her distress. However, our formulation acknowledges aspects of Molly's experience that, realistically, she has little control, or perhaps even conscious awareness, of: the influence of systems around her and the implicit structuring of her emotional experience that have developed through her life. We understand the concept of repeating patterns to be common to all three models to varying degrees. Where the CBT model might describe the activation of core beliefs and implementation of maladaptive coping strategies, systemic theory would see the interaction of one's expectations and that of the system as eliciting ineffective and repetitive attempts to solve and rebalance. Lastly, psychodynamic theory might describe the replication of unconscious relational structures in the present. Across these conceptualisations lies a similar goal and point of core congruence: to identify core beliefs and schemas, observe interactional patterns in systems, or bring the unconscious into conscious awareness. Integrating three theoretical positions is helpful here in reminding us (as Molly's hypothetical therapists) that to imply that complete control over one's experience can ever be gained would be unrealistic and unhelpful.

11.4.3 Meaning in Practice

In practice, by helping Molly to understand and manage these somewhat less directly controllable influences on her mental health, at the same time as directly targeting distress through CBT techniques, we would support her to consider what is and is not within her control to change. Steele, van der Hart, and Nijenhuis (2001) suggest that mental health is associated with an individual's capacity to integrate events, as this enables distributed attention and the possibility of reflective thought and action. Our understanding of integrating these different theories for clients with complex problems – like Molly – would mirror Steele et al.'s (2001) suggestion that a broader appreciation of the factors influencing behaviour and change will be supportive of personal integration and mental health.

11.4.4 Intervention Objectives

Intervention using an integrative approach requires integration of techniques reflecting models used in the formulation; in this case, cognitive, behavioural, systemic, and psychodynamic. There is no one way of organising and delivering the techniques, just as there was no one way of integrating and building the formulation. However, there are empirically supported approaches to draw upon as described in previous chapters, and, of particular relevance to integration, within the 'common factors' literature. The primary focus of 'common factors' based efficacy research has been to specify empirically supported aspects of the therapeutic relationship (e.g., Hardy, Cahill, & Barkham, 2007; Norcross, 2011).

Although empirically supported aspects of the therapeutic relationship are too wide-ranging to fully consider here, we highlight a few key objectives for establishing an effective alliance with Molly. Better outcomes have been associated with clients understanding their role and that of the therapist in the work, as well as clients and therapists having hopeful expectations of achieving success (Hardy et al., 2007). Clients' intentions and motivation for change have also been linked to more positive results (Hardy et al., 2007). Hence our initial approach to working with Molly would focus on developing an effective therapeutic relationship in which we could agree on goals for change that seem desirable, meaningful, and manageable to both Molly and us.

11.4.5 Intervention Plan

Whilst 'pure-form' theoretical approaches point in particular directions to define appropriate goals, the flexibility of our integrative approach would draw on responsiveness from Molly and aspects of the formulation that fit with her perspectives to facilitate closer collaboration. As agreement about goals and collaborating in an alliance to achieve these has been linked to positive therapeutic outcomes (Norcross, 2011), psychoeducation about the process of therapy and relevant aspects of the formulation could help Molly understand what to expect and how this might be achieved. We know that Molly wants to feel "better", "more confident" and the "opposite" of how she currently feels. Once more clearly specified, these goals might be achievable through developing alternative coping skills – enhancing her abilities to challenge unhelpful thinking patterns, and to choose less damaging behaviours when she is struggling. Through initial attempts to directly target her immediate distress, we might both try to address issues of risk inherent in her presentation, as well as begin to gauge the extent of her ability to respond to CBT-type interventions.

One of Molly's stated goals is to "make everyone proud", but this needs exploration as her history suggests she might be overly focused on pleasing others at personal cost. Our formulation has also highlighted a repeated pattern of failing to 'achieve' to the level expected by those around her, so a CBT skills focus in the work has the potential to evoke a familiar story of failure within the therapy. Our understanding of the systemic aspects of this case would become particularly relevant in such circumstances and we might aim to help Molly to understand the influence of the systems around her in developing this narrative. If it was possible to help Molly to distinguish her systems' goals from more personal goals, this might usefully support her motivation for and expectancies of change. She might choose to adjust her narrative about her needs and abilities, rather than simply aiming to directly change problematic thoughts and behaviours.

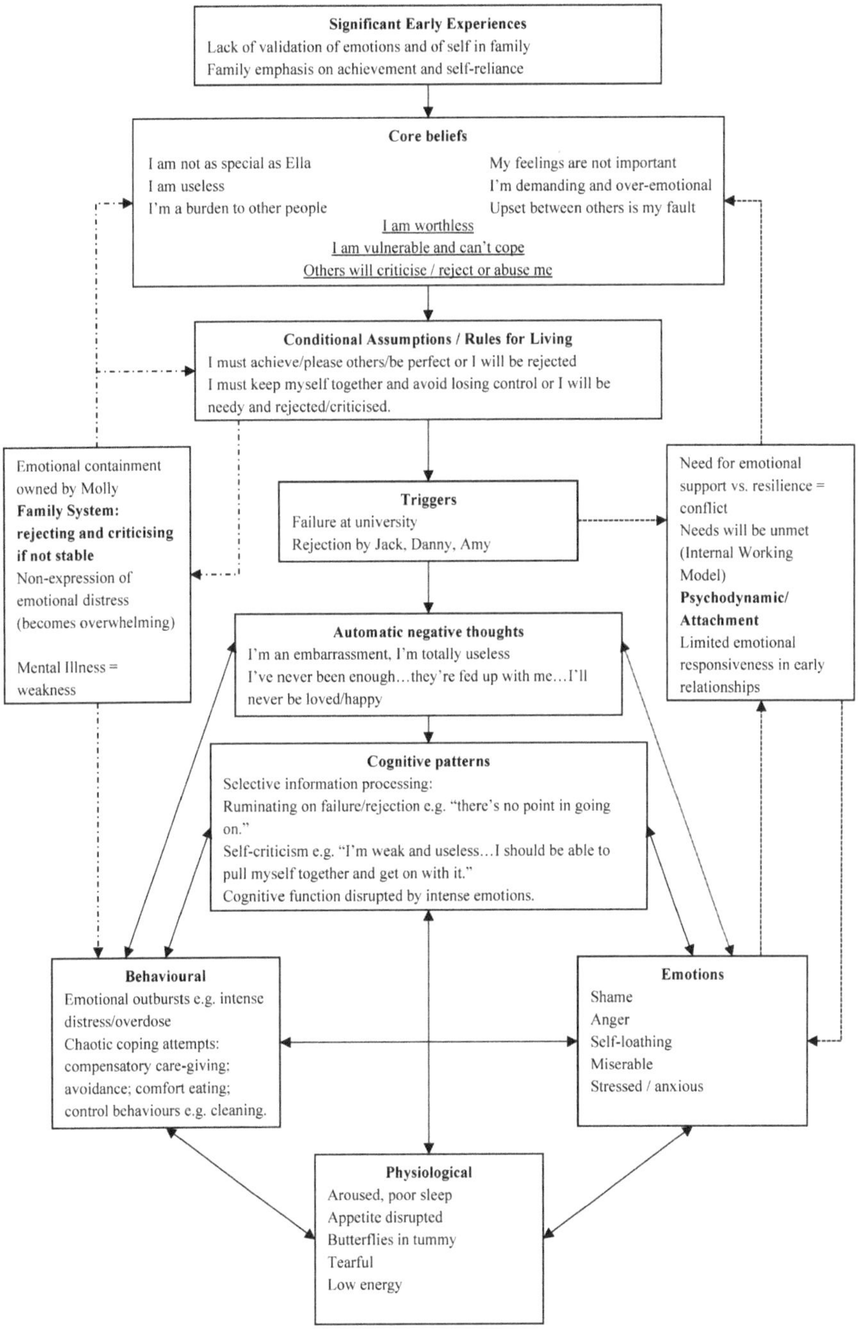

Figure 11.2: Diagrammatic integrative formulation

Empathy, positive regard, and affirmation are also associated with therapeutic success, although therapists' expressions of these need adjustment to fit particular clients' needs (Norcross, 2011). As Molly is used to keeping others at a distance and her home life 'lacked warmth', we expect she will not be able to receive warmth and empathy without a degree of internal conflict. Receiving something so needed but lacking in her life could serve as a painful reminder of what she missed and stimulate a greater sense of neediness, which she 'hates' in herself already. Gentle enquiry into how Molly experiences small offerings of attuned care could facilitate exploration of the significance of her unmet needs in her experience of relationships generally. Additionally, findings from neuroscience suggest that adult experiences of empathic responding in the therapeutic relationship can foster trust and promote implicit emotion regulation abilities (Wilkinson, 2010). Such work could become more of a focus if Molly struggles to take conscious control of creating change.

In summary then, we would plan to start work with Molly by building the relationship, being aware of the attachment issues and potential conflict highlighted throughout. Realistically, this development of attachment and modelling by the therapist, as well as the provision of safety, will need to run throughout the therapy. CBT tools will be utilised, including shared building of her formulation, before moving to consider use of techniques like cognitive restructuring and behavioural experiments, some of which would test the system (family and workplace) in which Molly resides. These in turn will help begin to challenge Molly's IWM. The last phase of work would probably focus on the system, predominantly the family. Educating Molly and refining our shared understanding of her behaviours and attempts to maintain the stability of the system will allow her to build more functional strategies of responding in the future. In actuality, the therapist and Molly will consider the best steps to take at each point through the therapeutic journey.

11.4.6 Effectiveness

Measuring effectiveness in this case is open to many possibilities and it is important to consider in an ongoing manner, so that the therapist can respond to and adjust strategies or techniques that are not working. Within the CBT aspects of the work, one might consider effectiveness as a shift in long held cognitions (that cause distress) and use of new behaviours. Given we believe that the system impacts upon Molly's belief systems, changing some of these beliefs will be unlikely to happen if the system is not considered or challenged. CBT will also provide Molly with cognitive skills she can use to better manage the scenarios that she faces; such as appropriate emotional expression, practiced and not rejected throughout therapy. Thus we could note the number of new skills Molly develops. We could also consider effectiveness through Molly's attendance or contributions in sessions, completion of tasks outside of the session, or a growth in confidence. We could notice the negative language about self that Molly uses and how this changes over the course of therapy and/or gather weekly ratings of mood or therapeutic alliance. Ultimately, however, all three models would allow consideration of Molly's goals and how far she has achieved them as a sensible way of considering outcome. Perhaps most telling will be change in the levels of distress Molly reports over time, as well as whether she feels "different" to how she felt at the beginning of her journey. We must of course consider the possibility that her original goals may change throughout therapy, thus her goal to "make everyone proud" may come to reflect a more flexible and achievable goal.

David M Gresswell

11.5 Integrative Formulation: Critical Commentary

Helpfully, this chapter not only illustrates the shortcomings of an "integrative approach" but also the shortcomings of CBT, "systemic", and psychodynamic approaches. As the authors indicate, the evidence-base for integrative approaches (as opposed to the individual components of relationships, techniques, and so forth) is weak. However, putting that issue to one side, the approach also invites a somewhat uncommitted and undisciplined approach to formulation – specifically: When the going gets tough, switch models.

To begin with the CBT model that the authors open with, the longitudinal approach to formulation illustrated in Figure 11.1 falls into several "post-Beckian" traps: including lack of internal consistency, lack of nuance, an incoherent model of emotion, and overlooking the contingencies that maintain the behaviour. Examining the so-called "core beliefs", these are clearly inconsistent with the conditional assumptions and behaviour – if Molly truly believes she is useless how can she also believe that she must (can) please others and that she can avoid criticism? Why does she seek employment and so forth? The issue here is partly one of nuance: Surely Molly's "belief" that she is useless varies according to context and could be rephrased into something more consistent with the rest of the formulation and her actual behaviour?

Turning to the conceptualisation of emotion, Beck started off by attempting to explain depression; however, in the approach illustrated in this chapter, we can see the same core beliefs, conditional assumptions, triggers, etc. being used to explain five emotions (specifically: shame, anger, self-loathing, miserableness, and stress) all at the same time – clearly this isn't going to work. The problem is compounded by the theoretical incoherence of the model of emotion: In this formulation the five emotions listed in the "Emotions" box are separate from, but interact with, physiology, behaviour, and cognition. If emotion is independent of cognition, behaviour, and physiology then, phenomenologically, what is it?

Finally the formulation model does not consider the external variables (contingencies) that maintain the behaviours in question – e.g., if you are prone to emotional outbursts you will get different responses from someone who is generally reserved. This is a fundamental flaw in the CBT approach to an A:B:C formulation. Beck and colleagues effectively changed it from an operant Stimulus:Response:Stimulus (S:R:S) model – in which “A” is a Stimulus (the trigger for a behavioural sequence), “B” is a Response (everything the person does), and “C” is another Stimulus (the consequences contingent on the behaviour that influence it in some way) – to, in effect, an incomplete S:R1:R2 model – in which “A” is still a trigger, but the “B” (R1) now represents some cognitive processing (typically called “beliefs” in many CBT texts), and the “C” (R2) represents some form of additional “emotional” response to R1. The contingencies which follow on from R1 and R2 have been unhelpfully dropped from the analysis. Rather than address these issues in a disciplined fashion, the archetypal integrative psychologist merely stumbles, half acknowledges the problem, and flips models – in this case, the authors shift to a so-called “systemic approach”.

At the risk of sounding like a psychological Margaret Thatcher, there is no “system”; but, as is well illustrated here, simply a number of individuals (family members, fellow students, colleagues) reinforcing and punishing each other’s behaviour. There is no “systemic theory” illustrated in the chapter; but merely a description of the probable ways (based on history) in which Molly’s mother will, for example, punish some of Molly’s behaviours (thereby causing anxiety and suppressing the behaviour), ignore some other behaviours (contributing to extinction), and intermittently reinforce still others (thereby strengthening them). A thorough behavioural functional analysis would focus on these issues, consider who is influencing who through reciprocal reinforcement and on what schedules, and thereby actually inform the intervention.

Despite two attempts, the authors still consider the formulation incomplete because it does not consider the “unconscious...” In attempting to add an attachment-based interpretation of these unconscious processes, what is highlighted is that Molly’s expressions of anger have probably been punished in the past, and so she acts to suppress angry behaviour now to avoid expected punishment. It would seem highly unlikely that Molly is unaware of these processes given her description of her family life. The result of all this model changing and “integration” is the even more complicated “diagrammatic integrative formulation” illustrated in Figure 11.2, in which the inconsistencies and anomalies evident in the first formulation are not only perpetuated but are now supported by additional boxes: one on the left, with the term “family system” emboldened (which presumably describes how Molly’s family punish and reward her behaviour); and another on the right, which primarily contains “needs” and “Psychodynamic/attachment” issues. These boxes are attached to the initial Beckian formulation with broken lines and arrows – thereby adding the circular links beloved of systemic theorists. Nevertheless these circular links fail to show how the different components of the formulation actually and specifically interact with each other.

Although the authors make the point that they "cannot imagine the 'cold war' (between competing ideologies) as described by Norcross", we think their chapter (inadvertently) makes an argument for a return to those days and to the disciplined thinking of the advocates of the different ideologies. For us, the chapter affirms the need to teach trainee psychological practitioners a holistic model of human behaviour (such as radical behaviourism) and then train them to develop, apply, and rigorously test a comprehensive and theoretically-informed functional analysis in a disciplined and committed fashion. The alternative would seem to be to create a generation of psychological practitioners who are 'jacks of several trades and masters of none' – surely the rational thing to do when things go wrong is not to change models at the first opportunity, but to really think about the new data gained, question why the initial formulation hypotheses have been disproved, re-work the formulation, and then test it again?

Louise Braham & Sharron Smith

11.6 Author Response

There appears to be an essential difference in philosophy underpinning an Integrative perspective and this critique's perspective. Where we see drawing on a variety of explanatory models as an aid to appreciating the complexity of factors shaping Molly's distress, this critique characterises her experience as reducible to stimuli and responses. We reject the notion that an Integrative approach advocates switching models when one gets stuck. The approach advocates a systematic choosing of aspects of models that allow integration and the development of a fuller picture of a range of mechanisms contributing to an individual's psychological life. Integration should be a well-considered process informed by reflection on theory, literature, the client, and their experience.

Given the complexity of human beings generally and Molly's difficulties specifically, we accept that the diagrammatic formulation and verbal account in this chapter were necessarily heavily summarised and consequently limited in their precision. However, in practice, a more nuanced formulation could be generated through collaboration with Molly and focusing on specific goals.

The critical commentary authors highlight that Molly's belief about being useless is inconsistent with a belief that she must and can please others. Whilst it might appear inconsistent, as humans are complex organisms they are able to hold more than one view or belief, even those that seem contradictory. In this case, the beliefs are opposite ends of the same continuum, so moving between 'useless' and 'pleasing' (i.e., being useful to others) is part of Molly's struggle and distress. Equally, although it is complicated to account for multiple emotional experiences, distress is rarely (if ever) one-dimensional and emotion labels can encapsulate experiences in a way that is ideally both meaningful and containing for clients.

What Molly might be aware of or not is another question raised by this critique and we accept the concept of 'the unconscious' as potentially problematic. We appreciate having the space here to highlight 'mentalization' (e.g., Fonagy, Gergely, Jurist, & Target, 2004), a concept that fits better with our intersubjective stance. Whilst 'the unconscious' implies awareness is simply not present, accounts of mentalization suggest individuals' reflective abilities are not constant but fluctuate according to context. Particularly for people considered 'personality disordered', non-reflective functioning is thought to dominate behaviour when there is conflict in relationships.

The critique offered is little more than a criticism of something that is not 'behavioural'. Potentially, our formulation could be broadened to include a behavioural perspective, but we wonder how Molly might receive such an account. Another apparently fundamental difference between the critical commentary and our Integrative perspective concerns the position of the client in relation to formulation. Rather than privileging an account that we regard as technically 'the correct one', we aim to use formulations that are meaningful and engaging for our clients, as well as theoretically coherent. We believe that psychological practitioners should be trained in a number of theories and models (in a pure way) so they can ultimately utilise skills of analysis and integration to make models that fit individual clients.

References

Bowlby, J. (1969). *Attachment and loss: Vol. 1. Attachment.* London: Penguin.

Bowlby, J. (1973). *Attachment and loss: Vol. 2. Separation: Anxiety and anger.* London: Penguin.

Brooks-Harris, J. E. (2008). *Integrative multitheoretical psychotherapy.* New York: Houghton Mifflin.

Dollard, J., & Miller, N. E. (1950). *Personality and psychotherapy: An analysis in terms of learning, thinking and culture.* New York: McGraw-Hill.

Fonagy, P., Gergely, G., Jurist, E., & Target, M. (2004). *Affect regulation, mentalization and the development of the self.* London: Karnac.

Gilbert, M., & Orlans, V. (2011). *Integrative therapy: 100 key points and techniques.* Hove: Routledge.

Grencavage, L. M., & Norcross, J. C. (1990). Where are the commonalities among the therapeutic common factors? *Professional Psychology: Research and Practice, 21*(5), 372-378.

Hardy, G., Cahill, J., & Barkham, M. (2007). Active ingredients of the therapeutic relationship that promote client change: A research perspective. In P. Gilbert & R. L. Leahy (Eds.), *The therapeutic relationship in the cognitive behavioral psychotherapies* (pp. 24-42). London: Routledge.

Ingram, B. L. (2006). *Clinical case formulations: Matching the integrative treatment plan to the client.* Hoboken, NJ: John Wiley & Sons.

McLeod, J. (2009). *An introduction to counselling* (4th ed.). Buckingham: Open University Press.

Norcross, J. C. (2005). A primer on psychotherapy integration. In J. C. Norcross & M. R. Goldfried (Eds.), *Handbook of psychotherapy integration* (2nd ed., pp. 3-23). New York: Oxford.

Norcross, J. C. (2011). *Psychotherapy relationships that work* (2nd ed.). New York: Oxford University Press.

Prochaska, J. O. (1979). *Systems of psychotherapy: A transtheoretical analysis.* Homewood, IL: Dorsey Press.

Prochaska, J. O., & Norcross, J. C. (2010). *Systems of psychotherapy: A transtheoretical analysis* (7th ed.). Pacific Grove, CA: Brooks/Cole.

Rosenzweig, S. (1936). Some implicit common factors in diverse methods of psychotherapy. *American Journal of Orthopsychiatry, 6*(3), 412-415.

Ryle, A. (1995). *Cognitive Analytic Therapy: Developments in theory and practice.* Chichester: John Wiley & Sons.

Steele, K., van der Hart, O., & Nijenhuis, E. R. (2001). Dependency in the treatment of complex posttraumatic stress disorder and dissociative disorders. *Journal of Trauma & Dissociation, 2*(4), 79-116.

Stern, D. (1985). *The interpersonal world of the infant: A view from psychoanalysis and development psychology*. London: Karnac.

Tracey, T. J., Lichtenberg, J. W., Goodyear, R. K., Claiborn, C. D., & Wampold, B. E. (2003). Concept mapping of therapeutic common factors. *Psychotherapy Research, 13*(4), 401-413.

Wachtel, P. L. (1977). *Psychoanalysis and behavior therapy: Toward an integration*. New York: Basic Books.

Wampold, B. E. (2001). *The great psychotherapy debate: Models, methods, and findings*. Mahwah, NJ: Erlbaum.

Wampold, B. E., Mondin, G. W., Moody, M., Stich, F., Benson, K., & Ahn, H. (1997). A meta-analysis of outcome studies comparing bona fide psychotherapies: Empiricially," all must have prizes.". *Psychological Bulletin, 122*(3), 203-215.

Weerasekera, P. (1996). *Multiperspective case formulation: A step towards treatment integration*. Malabar, FL: Krieger Publishing Company.

Wilkinson, M. (2010). *Changing minds in therapy: Emotion, attachment, trauma and neurobiology*. London: Norton.

Young, J. E., Klosko, J. S., & Weishaar, M. (2003). *Schema Therapy: A practitioner's guide*. New York: Guilford Publications.

Contributors

Kerry Beckley is a Consultant Forensic Clinical Psychologist in Lincolnshire, UK, working with community forensic services and the National Probation Service. She is a trainer and supervisor in Schema Therapy, and is the current chair of the Group Schema Therapy Committee (International Society of Schema Therapy). She graduated from Southampton University in 2002, after completing her doctoral thesis evaluating the use of the Young Schema Questionnaire (YSQ) with Adolescents. Her interests are in the application of Schema Therapy to forensic populations and individuals with personality difficulties, and she has published and presented widely in this area.

Louise Braham is a Consultant Clinical Forensic Psychologist working in Forensic Services in Nottinghamshire. She also holds the position of Senior Clinical Tutor on the Trent Doctorate in Clinical Psychology. Louise has a keen interest in the application of psychology to broader mental health services and, although trained in a number of applications (such as schema therapy, EMDR, CBT), works in an integrative way. She has an interest in neuropsychology, and holds an MSc in Clinical Neuropsychology. Louise has published (in books and peer reviewed journals) on a range of topics in the clinical and forensic fields.

Roger Bretherton is a Clinical Psychologist and Senior Lecturer in the School of Psychology at the University of Lincoln, UK. He received his doctorate in Clinical Psychology in 1999 and worked in adult mental health services in the NHS for over a decade. His qualifications cover a wide range of therapeutic approaches, including: Existential Psychotherapy; Dialectical Behaviour Therapy; Sensorimotor Psychotherapy; and Positive Psychology. His recent research focuses on character strengths such as gratitude, compassion, courage, and humility, and their relationship to psychological wellbeing.

Angela Cooper is a Chartered Clinical Psychologist working in adult secondary mental health services in South West Yorkshire, UK. She is about to embark on a 2-year work placement for the Centre of Emotions and Health in Halifax, Nova Scotia, Canada, where she will work using Intensive Short-term Dynamic Psychotherapy (ISTDP) with people experiencing medically unexplained symptoms and chronic pain. She graduated from the Trent Doctorate in Clinical Psychology, UK, in 2011 after completing her doctoral thesis investigating whether self-compassion can moderate risk factors such as shame and self-criticism in a trauma population. She has an interest in the process and mechanisms of change within psychotherapy, particularly how to maximise therapeutic effectiveness, and has published in this area.

Vanessa Dale-Hewitt is a Clinical Psychologist working in perinatal psychiatry in Nottinghamshire, UK. She also holds the position of Academic Tutor on the Trent Doctorate in Clinical Psychology. She graduated from Sheffield University, in 2007, after completing her doctoral thesis investigating attentional patterns in women who developed post-traumatic stress following childbirth. She has a longstanding interest in cognitive, attachment, and Compassion Focused Therapy and treatment, and has published in this area.

Danielle De Boos is a Clinical Psychologist working in Mental Health Services for Older People in Nottinghamshire, UK. She also holds the position of Clinical Tutor and Lecturer in Clinical Psychology on the Trent Doctoral Training Programme at the University of Nottingham, UK. Her doctoral thesis applied Interpretative Phenomenological Analysis to explore diagnostic processes in UK minority ethnic groups.

Nima G Moghaddam is a Chartered Clinical Psychologist and HCPC-registered Practitioner Psychologist. He works on the Trent Doctoral Programme in Clinical Psychology at the University of Lincoln, UK. He has an enduring interest in the pragmatic application of contextual psychological theories to describe, predict, and influence everyday behaviour.

Aidan J P Hart is a registered Clinical and Forensic Psychologist, and a Senior Lecturer in psychology at the University of Lincoln, UK. Aidan qualified as a Clinical Psychologist in 2006, after completing his doctorate and clinical training at the University of Sheffield, UK. He has a long standing interest in behavioural analysis, behavioural theory, and third-wave approaches to therapy.

David L Dawson is a Chartered Clinical Psychologist and works on the Trent Doctoral Programme in Clinical Psychology at the University of Lincoln, UK. He is interested in the development and application of broad psychological theories and technologies which place significant emphasis on the prediction and influence of psychological events and behaviour.

David M Gresswell is a Clinical Psychologist working in forensic services in Lincolnshire, UK. He is also the Lincoln-based programme director of the Trent Doctorate in Clinical Psychology. He graduated from Leicester University, UK, in 1988. He has a long-standing interest in radical behaviourism and classical conditioning.

Chris Irons is a Clinical Psychologist and a board member of the Compassionate Mind Foundation. In his clinical work, he uses Compassion Focused Therapy (CFT) and he regularly presents to academic, professional, and lay audiences on CFT and, more broadly, the science of compassion. He is interested in the theoretical and clinical developments and adaptations of CFT as a science-based psychotherapeutic approach.

Rohan Naidoo is a Clinical Psychologist working at a social enterprise called Compass Wellbeing in London, UK. There he offers NHS funded assessment and brief experiential dynamic psychotherapy for primary care patients. After studying politics and philosophy, he converted to psychology and graduated from the Trent Doctorate in Clinical Psychology in 2011. His doctoral thesis explored the relationship between personal identity, experiential avoidance, and therapeutic change. He has a special interest in the interface between psychology and philosophy, focussing especially on the relationships between selfhood, morality, and wellbeing.

Mike Rennoldson is a Clinical Psychologist working with adults with blood cancers in Sheffield, UK. He also holds the position of Academic Tutor on the Trent Doctorate in Clinical Psychology. He graduated from Plymouth University, UK, in 2006 after completing his doctoral thesis investigating the use of social support by men with colorectal cancer. He has a longstanding interest in social approaches to psychological care, having also trained as a systemic practitioner and published in this area.

Rachel Sabin-Farrell is a Clinical Psychologist working within adult mental health services in Nottinghamshire, UK. She also holds the position of Senior Academic Tutor on the Trent Doctorate in Clinical Psychology. She graduated from Sheffield University, UK, in 2000 after completing a doctoral thesis investigating the impact on UK mental health workers of working with traumatised clients. She has a longstanding interest in the psychological effects of trauma and abuse, both clinically and in her teaching/research activities, and has published papers in this area. She has also trained in the treatment of trauma using Eye Movement Desensitisation and Reprocessing (EMDR) and Sensorimotor Psychotherapy, and has supervised research in both of these therapeutic approaches.

Thomas Schröder is the Nottingham-based programme director of the Trent Doctorate in Clinical Psychology. After working for 25 years as a consultant in a multidisciplinary psychotherapy service, his current clinical role centres on helping people suffering from traumatic stress. His research interests include the professional development of therapists, difficulties in psychotherapeutic practice, and self-conscious emotions in psychological therapy and supervision. He is a past president of the UK chapter of the Society for Psychotherapy Research, a Trustee of the Compassionate Mind Foundation, and a Senior Fellow of the Institute of Mental Health.

Sharron Smith is a Clinical Psychologist supporting adults with serious and enduring mental health problems in Nottinghamshire, UK. She also holds the position of Senior Clinical Tutor for Lincolnshire on the Trent Doctorate in Clinical Psychology.

She qualified as a Clinical Psychologist in 2000 after training at Leeds University, UK, and completing her doctoral thesis exploring psychological adaptation in later life. She has a longstanding interest in Integration and completed a Masters in Integrative Psychotherapy with the Sherwood Institute in 2009.

Ray St. Ledger is a Clinical Psychologist, Forensic Psychologist, and Neuropsychologist. He works for the NHS in Wakefield Prison with individuals with diagnoses of personality disorder and learning disabilities, and in Coventry with the neuropsychological rehabilitation team. He lectures on the Clinical Psychology Doctoral Programme at the University of Sheffield, UK. He qualified as a Clinical Psychologist in 1990 and is interested in the neuropsychology of motivation and self-regulation.

Anna Tickle is a Clinical Psychologist working with adults with intellectual disabilities in Nottinghamshire, UK. She also holds the position of Academic Research Tutor on the Trent Doctorate in Clinical Psychology. Since qualifying as a Clinical Psychologist in 2009, Anna has undertaken further training in family therapy and became a systemic practitioner in 2012.

List of Figures

List of Tables

Index

FSC
www.fsc.org
MIX
Papier | Fördert gute Waldnutzung
FSC® C083411

Kolibri 360 GmbH
Ferdinand-Jühlke-Straße 7
99095 Erfurt, Deutschland
produktsicherheit@kolibri360.de